Dr Atkins

New

Carbohydrate

Counter

Dr Atkins
New
Carbohydrate
Counter

**Companion to the
international bestseller,
Dr Atkins New Diet Revolution**

Dr Robert C Atkins

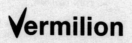

1 3 5 7 9 10 8 6 4 2

First published in the US in 2002 by M. Evans and Company
First published in the United Kingdom in 2003 by
Vermilion, an imprint of Ebury Press
Random House UK Ltd.
Random House
20 Vauxhall Bridge Road
London SW1V 2SA

Random House Australia (Pty) Limited
20 Alfred Street, Milsons Point, Sydney,
New South Wales 2061, Australia

Random House New Zealand Limited
18 Poland Road, Glenfield,
Auckland 10, New Zealand

Random House (Pty) Limited
Endulini, 5A Jubilee Road, Parktown 2193, South Africa

Random House UK Limited Reg. No. 954009
www.randomhouse.co.uk
Papers used by Vermilion are natural, recyclable products
made from wood grown in sustainable forests.

A CIP catalogue record is available for this book from the
British Library.

ISBN: 0091889472

Printed and bound in Great Britain by
Bookmarque Ltd, Croydon. Surrey

Contents

Foreword

Why Publish a New Edition?

In the six years since this book was first published, more and more people have embraced the idea of limiting carbohydrate intake for weight control – as well as overall good health. Numerous scientific studies have corroborated the logic of the Atkins philosophy. Meanwhile, as the twin epidemics of obesity and diabetes have picked up pace, mainstream health professionals are increasingly realizing that achieving a healthy weight is not just a matter of cutting back on fat and calories. There is a growing awareness that sugar, white flour, trans fats and the junk foods made with them are a large part of the problem.

To make this book more useful, we've made a host of improvements:

• **Use of a new software program.** This system enables us to provide more precise nutritional information.

• **More data.** We provide not just grams of carbohydrate, but also Net Carbs. These are the only carbs you need to count when you do Atkins because they exclude carbohydrates such as fibre and sugar alcohol, which have a minimal impact on blood sugar. Although there is no need to count calories if you are counting carbs, many people find it psychologically gratifying to know how many calories they are consuming, so we have added them as well.

- **More controlled carb foods.** Bagels made with soya flour and pancake mixes made with wheat gluten and starch-resistant maize contain a fraction of the carbs found in white flour versions. Comparable offerings among breakfast cereals, breads, muffins, crackers and even pasta allow you to enjoy such traditional foods without overloading on sugar and starch.

- **Other new products.** We also have added or increased our inclusion of soya products, pastas made from grains other than wheat and brands such as Newman's Own and Far East that now are commonly found on grocery shelves.

- **More vegetables.** This section has been considerably amplified, acknowledging the importance of these most nutrient-dense carbohydrates, so you can select those lowest in carbs.

- **More categories.** To make it easier for you to find what you are looking for, we've divided previous grouped food categories such as 'Desserts and Snacks' into two. Within categories, we've made entries more logical. Now, for example, pork loin and ham appear under a pork heading, instead of scattered alphabetically throughout an overall meat listing.

- **New sections.** These short chapters help with the practicalities of eating out. 'Dining Out' allows you to make informed choices among a wide variety of ethnic cuisines. 'Fast Foods' offers assistance in navigating the treacherous waters – carbwise – in such establishments. You'll learn how to estimate portions when you are not in your own kitchen in 'Portion Size Guidelines.'

This revised edition of *Dr Atkins New Carbohydrate Counter* is the perfect companion to the recently revised bestselling *Dr Atkins New Diet Revolution*, which reflects Dr Atkins' latest thinking and current terminology. The changes are not just linguistic. The name of Atkins Nutritional Approach™ (instead of the Atkins diet) reflects the fact that eating controlled carbohydrate foods is actually a prescription for a permanent healthy lifestyle. Seven new chapters clarify the Atkins approach, with twice as many references as the former edition, 100 brand new recipes and tips for making it easier than ever to follow the programme. You may also want to read *Dr Atkins Quick & Easy Cookbook*, written with Veronica Atkins. For more information on these books and the Atkins Nutritional Approach™, go to *www.atkinscenter.com*.

Introduction

Congratulations! If you've purchased this book, you've made a decision to pursue the controlled carbohydrate path to weight control. But you may not yet realize that you will likely also enjoy improved energy and better health by following the Atkins Nutritional Approach™.

We know you can't wait to get started. If you are already limiting your carbohydrate intake, you already understand that it's a proven way to once and for all take control of your weight. But Atkins is much more. *Dr Atkins New Diet Revolution* fully explains the four principles upon which it is based. But in brief, by doing Atkins for a lifetime, you can:

- **Lose weight.** Achieving optimal weight is an important component of good health.
- **Maintain that weight loss.** The problem with most diets is not that they don't work, but that they don't last. When doing Atkins, you gradually add back carb foods until you reach the level of carbohydrate intake that allows you to maintain a healthy weight.
- **Achieve good health.** When doing Atkins, nutritional needs are met with wholesome, whole foods.
- **Lay the groundwork for disease prevention.** Controlling

carbs lowers insulin levels, which lowers risk factors for chronic diseases, including heart disease, hypertension, diabetes and certain cancers.

Understanding these principles makes it clear that Atkins is not just a diet that you start when you have a few pounds to lose and stop when you reach your goal. Four phases (described on pages 16–17) enable you to gradually change your eating habits, resulting in a lifetime of slimness. Doing Atkins also allows you to establish an eating programme that is individually tailored to your needs, based on your age, gender, metabolism and level of physical activity.

Carbohydrates Versus Calories and Fat

The reason that millions of copies of *New Diet Revolution* have been sold and that millions of individuals swear by Atkins is very simple: It works. Even if you've failed on low-fat diets, once you understand that the real culprit is an over-reliance on carbohydrate foods, particularly those full of sugar, refined flour and other processed ingredients, you are on the path to success. In the last two decades, three things have happened:

- Our culture has been obsessed with dietary fat.
- Low-fat and fat-free products proliferated – many of them junk foods loaded with white flour, sugar and other nutrient-deficient ingredients.
- Nonetheless, by eating these foods we have become fatter than ever.

The culprit is not fat per se; it's the over-consumption of carbohydrates. Obviously, counting calories and restricting fat intake has not worked. The average individual now consumes upwards of 300g of carbs a day, far too much for most people to metabolize (burn as energy). When you eat foods high in carbs, your body converts them to glucose, or blood sugar, which is released into your blood stream. Your pancreas then releases the hormone insulin, which transports the glucose to your cells. Whatever is not used for energy is stored as fat.

When blood glucose levels become elevated, the pancreas responds with a flood of insulin. Keep this up for years and your body can become incapable of utilizing the insulin efficiently. This metabolic disorder, called insulin resistance or hyper-insulimia, can be a precursor to diabetes. Being overweight, particularly very overweight, raises the risk of developing this condition. Insulin is known as the fat-producing hormone so excess insulin can lead to excessive fat. Fortunately, the solution to excessive insulin production is simple: Control carbohydrate intake.

A Metabolic Switch

The Atkins approach is fundamentally different to the low-fat approach to weight loss. Both carbohydrate and fat provide fuel for the body's energy needs. If carbohydrate is available, the body burns it as fuel first, but burning fat is also perfectly natural and safe. Switch your body from a glucose metabolism to a mostly fat metabolism, and you burn your body fat for energy instead of storing it. It is crucial that you understand that it's not simply *dietary* fat that makes you fat. Rather, it's excess carbohydrates, especially in the form of sugar, white flour and other starches – found in breads, pasta and potatoes and in almost all over-processed convenience foods and snacks.

Where Carbs Lurk

When you do Atkins, eating proteins, healthy fats and nutrient-dense carbohydrates helps stabilize your blood sugar so you don't get ravenously hungry or depleted of energy a few hours after eating. Most of us are unfamiliar with the sources of carbohydrates and their relative merits. In fact, many people think that only grains and sweets are carbohydrate foods and don't realize that they are found in milk, fruits and even vegetables. That's why this *Carbohydrate Gram Counter* is of immediate help in two important ways.

First, success in doing Atkins is dependent upon accurately calculating the carbohydrate grams consumed each day. To do this with ease, you need a handy reference guide so that your decisions are based on facts, not assumptions. Secondly, although manufactured foods carry a Nutrition Facts Panel mandated by the Food and Drug Administration, it can still be difficult to ascertain the actual Net Carbohydrate gram count of each food. The panel lists total grams of carbohydrates as well as the grams of dietary fibre. Subtract the dietary fibre from the total and you will have a rough idea of the Net Carbs, although this figure does not usually factor in sugar alcohol and definitely not glycerine, which have minimal impact on blood sugar. Moreover, if a label lists 0g of carbohydrate, it can actually be as high as 0.99g. It is also important to check the serving size upon which the calculations are based. You may find that a single serving is considerably smaller than the portion you are actually eating. Still, the Nutritional Panel information is a valuable adjunct to this carb gram counter and it is worth getting in the habit of reading food labels. They are a great way to become aware of the staggering amount of sugar in many foods. In the near future, these labels are expected to include trans fats broken out from the total fat. At this time, the only way to ascertain if trans fats are in a food is to search the list of ingredients for hydrogenated fat or partially hydrogenated fat.

It's important that you understand that we have included foods in the *Carbohydrate Gram Counter* that are not recommended on the Atkins Nutritional Approach™ so you can compare them with foods more appropriate to doing Atkins. Please also understand that a book of this size cannot be comprehensive. Although it is impossible to list every product or every flavour of each product, we have provided enough basic information so that (in concert with Nutritional Panel information) you can guesstimate the carb counts for specific items not listed herein.

Let me leave you with three more pieces of important advice. Be sure to drink at least eight 250ml glasses of water a day to flush out your system and avoid dehydration or constipation. No matter what eating plan you choose to follow, a good multivitamin/mineral supplement ensures you get the recommended daily intake of all nutrients. And to complement and speed your weight loss, be sure to get plenty of exercise.

My *Carbohydrate Counter* will make it easier than ever to do Atkins and I have every confidence that the changes in this edition will make it even more useful and user friendly.

—ROBERT C. ATKINS, M.D.

A Brief Look at the Four Phases of the Atkins Nutritional Approach™

1. Induction: This initial phase, the most restrictive of carbohydrates, jump-starts weight loss. You eat no more than 20g of Net Carbs per day, which translates into roughly 3 small handfuls of salad greens and other non-starchy veggies. You can eat liberal amounts of protein (meats, fish, poultry, eggs) and healthy fats. Atkins is not a licence to gorge. When you're hungry, eat the amount that makes you feel satisfied but not stuffed. Stay on Induction for a minimum of two weeks.

2. Ongoing Weight Loss: When you move to OWL, you deliberately slow your weight loss as you introduce more variety in nutrient-dense carbohydrate foods. So long as weight loss continues, you gradually increase your carb intake in the following manner: Week one, eat 25g of carbs per day; week two, move to 30g of carbs per day, and so forth, until weight loss stalls. Then back down to the previous level. This threshold is known as your Critical Carbohydrate Level for Losing (CCLL).

Choose your additional carbs wisely, first from vegetables low in carbohydrates, then from other fresh, healthful, nutrient- and fibre-rich sources. Typical 5g increments include 10 Brazil nuts, half an avocado or 2tbs of green beans. Then add berries, which are lower in carbs than other fruits. Some individuals can add back legumes and whole grains, as well as other fruits. Typical daily tolerance levels range anywhere from 30g to 90g of carbohydrate. The more you exercise, the more carbs you can handle.

3. Pre-Maintenance: When your weight goal is in sight, you move to this phase and increase your daily carb allotment in 10g increments each week until weight loss slows to one or two pounds a month. This excessively slow pace is deliberate as you internalize eating habits that become part of a permanent lifestyle for weight maintenance.

4. Lifetime Maintenance: When you reach your goal weight, you are officially in this phase. Depending upon your age, gender, activity level and genetics, you could possibly consume anywhere from 90g to 120g – or even more – of carbs per day. This threshold is your Critical Carbohydrate Level for Maintenance (CCLM). Most people can occasionally eat modest portions of foods such as potatoes and other starchy vegetables, and regular (not controlled carb) wholewheat pasta and wholegrain bread without regaining weight. On the other hand, extremely metabolically resistant individuals may never be able to go beyond, say, 30g of carbs. No matter what your CCLM, for good health, continue to avoid white flour, sugar and all junk foods.

These four phases are fully described in *Dr Atkins New Diet Revolution*, along with lists of acceptable foods and suggested menus for each phase.

How to Use This Book

We made this book pocket-sized for a very good reason. It should travel with you to the supermarket, your place of work, to the finest restaurants and – without question – to fast food places. At home it will help you plan meals. Making up menus and a shopping list before you head off to the supermarket will keep you on track. Stick to your list and you will not be tempted by foods that don't belong in your meals – and in your house. You will find you can simply avoid certain grocery aisles full of carb-filled foods. This book may be small, but the import of its content is huge. Refer to it regularly and you will begin to understand how little things add up and how seemingly small changes can make a significant difference.

If you've been on low-fat diets, you've undoubtedly counted calories. You may have also counted grams of fat. With Atkins, you count grams of carbohydrate, a job made easy with this handy guide. Although we have provided information on fat, protein and calories for reference, the main thing you need to concern yourself with is a food's Net Carb count. These are the only carbs that count when you do Atkins. Unlike total carbs, they don't include the fibre, sugar alcohols and glycerine that have little impact on your blood sugar levels. (Also keep an eye on fibre content to ensure that you have adequate roughage in your diet. fibre also slows the entry of glucose into your blood stream, reducing blood sugar spikes and helps rid your body of cholesterol.)

Build your meals around protein foods such as meat, fish, poultry and eggs, vegetables and healthy fats such as olive oil and other monounsaturated fats. There is no need to restrict fat so long as you are controlling your carb intake. The one exception is trans fats, the hydrogenated oils found in most margarines and many packaged foods. Butter is a much healthier option. Check labels for trans fat and pass up anything that contains it. Your body is unable to process this unnatural fat.

Plan your daily or weekly menus by picking foods with low carbohydrate counts. But this is not just a numbers game: 20g of carbs from a jam doughnut do not equal 20g from three small handfuls of salad and other vegetables. Always select fresh, natural foods instead of refined, over-processed ones. Avoid anything made with white flour and sugar – and that includes most junk foods. When counting carbs, be sure to include those in snacks, beverages and artificial sweeteners.

The advice in this book is not meant to be a substitute for the advice of your personal physician. If you are embarking on a weight-loss programme, you should see your doctor first.

CAUTION: The advice offered in this book, although based on the author's experience with many thousands of patients, is not intended to be a substitute for the advice and counsel of your GP. If you are currently taking diuretics, insulin or oral diabetes medications, consult your physician before starting Atkins. You will need to reduce and then closely monitor your dosage as you lower your blood sugar level. People with severe kidney disease should not do Atkins. The weight loss phases of the Atkins Nutritional Approach are not appropriate for pregnant women and nursing mothers.

Portion Size Guidelines

Even on Atkins, it's important to be able to judge portion size, especially for higher carb foods. What does an 8cm slice look like? To help you recognize portions at a glance, we've created the following charts.

Bread and Grains

1 x 25g slice of bread	An index card
1 x 50g piece of Italian bread	A bar of soap
1 x 75g bagel	1 can of tuna
1 x 50g muffin	A cupcake wrapper

Fruits and Veggies

1 medium fruit	A tennis ball
1 small handful green salad	A fist
2 tablespoons cooked vegetables	A scoop of ice cream

Protein and Cheese

2 tablespoons peanut butter	Two teabags
75g beef, chicken or pork	A small pack of tissues or cigarettes
25g of cheese	A pair of dice
25g of nuts	Two ping pong balls or a small child's handful

Snacks and Desserts

25g of crisps

1 x 7.5cm piece of cake

A medium-sized handful

A small stack of business cards

Food Categories

BEVERAGES

Water is the most healthful beverage, but iced herbal teas and lemonades or limeades sweetened with a sugar substitute are suitable options for a change of pace. When you crave the flavour of fruit juice, purchase unsweetened concentrate (cranberry or passion fruit are good choices) in a health food shop and mix with sugar substitute and water or sparkling water. Some vegetable juices are a better bet: tomato juice has only 4 Net Carbs per 120ml and contains lycopene, an important antioxidant. Remember, when you are on the Lifetime Maintenance phase and decide to splurge on a Frappucino from Starbucks, you should think of it as a liquid dessert.

Though most alcoholic drinks – with the exception of sugar-laden fruit concoctions or drinks mixed with soda – are relatively low in carbs, they should be consumed in moderation. The body burns alcohol as a fuel before fat, so drinking alcohol slows down the fat-burning process. That said, after the Induction phase, an occasional glass of wine with dinner or a light beer is an acceptable part of a controlled carbohydrate lifestyle.

Food Item (Amount)	Carb (g)	Fibre (g)	Net Carbs (g)	Protein (g)	Fat (g)	Cals
Non-alcoholic Beverages						
CARBONATED/FIZZY DRINKS						
Cola (350ml)	38.7	0.0	38.7	0.0	0.0	153
Diet (350ml)	0.0	0.0	0.0	0.0	0.0	0
Ginger ale (350ml)	31.8	0.0	31.8	0.0	0.0	124
Grape (350ml)	41.7	0.0	41.7	0.0	0.0	160
Lemon-lime (350ml)	38.3	0.0	38.3	0.0	0.0	147
Root beer (350ml)	39.2	0.0	39.2	0.0	0.0	152
Sparkling water (350ml)	0.0	0.0	0.0	0.0	0.0	0
CHOCOLATE DRINKS						
Hot cocoa, Carnation, with marshmallows (1 pkt)	23.0	0.8	22.2	1.0	3.0	120
Hot cocoa, Nestlé, no sugar added (1 pkt)	8.4	0.8	7.6	4.3	0.4	55
Hot cocoa, Nestlé Rich Chocolate (1 pkt)	24.2	0.7	23.6	1.3	1.1	112
Nesquik Chocolate Drink (250ml)	33.0	1.0	32.0	7.0	8.0	230
COFFEE (see also Starbucks)						
Brewed (regular, decaf) (250ml)	1.0	0.0	1.0	0.2	0.0	5
Instant powder (1 tsp)	0.7	0.0	0.7	0.2	0.0	4
JUICES, FRUIT						
Apple (120ml)	14.5	0.1	14.4	0.1	0.1	58
Apricot nectar (120ml)	18.1	0.8	17.3	0.5	0.1	70
Cranberry juice cocktail, frozen, concentrate (30ml)	18.6	0.0	18.6	0.0	0.0	73
Cranberry juice cocktail, light,						

Food Item (Amount)	Carb (g)	Fibre (g)	Net Carbs (g)	Protein (g)	Fat (g)	Cals
Ocean Spray (120ml)	5.6	0.0	5.6	0.0	0.0	23
Cranberry juice cocktail (120ml)	18.2	0.1	18.1	0.0	0.1	72
Fruit punch (120ml)	14.8	0.1	14.6	0.0	0.0	58
Grape (120ml)	18.9	0.1	18.8	0.7	0.1	77
Grapefruit, sweetened (120ml)	13.9	0.1	13.8	0.7	0.1	58
Grapefruit, unsweetened (120ml)	11.1	0.1	11.0	0.6	0.1	47
Guava nectar (120ml)	19.0	1.0	18.0	0.2	0.1	74
Lemon (2 tbs)	2.6	0.1	2.5	0.1	0.0	8
Lime (2 tbs)	2.8	0.1	2.7	0.1	0.0	8
Mango nectar (120ml)	18.9	0.9	18.0	0.3	0.1	73
Orange, fresh (120ml)	12.9	0.3	12.7	0.9	0.3	56
Orange, from concentrate (120ml)	13.4	0.3	13.2	0.9	0.1	56
Passion fruit (120ml)	17.8	0.2	17.6	0.8	0.2	74
Peach nectar (120ml)	17.3	0.8	16.6	0.3	0.0	67
Pear nectar (120ml)	19.7	0.8	19.0	0.1	0.0	75
Pineapple (120ml)	17.2	0.3	17.0	0.4	0.1	70
Prune (120ml)	22.3	1.3	21.1	0.8	0.0	91
TROPICANA						
Grapefruit (100ml)	8	0.5	7.5	0.6	0	40
Multivitamins (100ml)	10.5	0.1	10.4	0.5	0	52
Original (100ml)	9	0.5	8.5	0.7	0	43
Tangerine Orange (120ml)	12.5	0.0	12.5	1.0	0.0	55
Tropics (100ml)	11	0	11	1	0	50

Food Item (Amount)	Carb (g)	Fibre (g)	Net Carbs (g)	Protein (g)	Fat (g)	Cals
GROVE FRESH (ORGANIC)						
Apple (100ml)	11.2	0.1	11.1	0.2	0	47
Apple and mango (100ml)	11.7	0.2	11.5	0.2	0	49
JUICES, VEGETABLE						
Carrot (120ml)	5.8	0.0	5.8	0.7	0.2	25
Tomato (120ml)	5.1	1.0	4.2	0.9	0.1	21
Vegetable juice cocktail (120ml)	5.5	1.0	4.5	0.8	0.1	23
MILK, FLAVOURED						
Banana	9.6	0	9.6	3.6	1.5	270
Chocolate (100g)	9.4	0	9.4	3.6	1.5	267
Strawberry (100g)	9.6	0	9.0	3.6	1.5	270
SNAPPLE						
Cranberry Raspberry drink, diet (250ml)	2.0	0.0	2.0	0.0	0.0	10
Kiwi Strawberry juice drink (250ml)	28.0	0.0	28.0	0.0	0.0	110
Tea, lemon, sweetened (250ml)	22.6	0.0	22.6	0.0	0.0	88
Tea, lemon, diet (250ml)	8.4	0.0	8.4	0.0	0.0	21
STARBUCKS						
Cappuccino, w/whole milk (350ml)	11.0	0.0	11.0	7.0	7.0	140
Frappuccino bottled (1 bottle)	37.0	0.0	37.0	7.0	3.5	200
Latte, iced, w/lowfat milk (350ml)	10.0	0.0	10.0	7.0	3.0	90
Latte, iced, w/whole milk (350ml)	10.0	0.0	10.0	6.0	6.0	120

Food Item (Amount)	Carb (g)	Fibre (g)	Net Carbs (g)	Protein (g)	Fat (g)	Cals
Latte, w/lowfat milk (350ml)	17.0	0.0	17.0	12.0	6.0	170
Latte, w/whole milk (350ml)	17.0	0.0	17.0	11.0	11.0	210
Mocha, w/whole milk (350ml)	33.0	1.0	32.0	12.0	20.0	340
Mocha Frappuccino (350ml)	44.0	0.0	44.0	6.0	3.0	230
TEA						
Brewed (250ml)	0.7	0.0	0.7	0.0	0.0	2
Herbal, brewed (250ml)	0.5	0.0	0.5	0.0	0.0	2
Iced, diet, Nestea (250ml)	1.2	0.0	1.2	0.0	0.0	3
Iced, sweetened, Nestea (250ml)	18.0	0.0	18.0	0.0	0.0	65
WATER (250ml)	0.0	0.0	0.0	0.0	0.0	0
Alcoholic Beverages						
BEER						
Beer (350ml)	13.2	0.7	12.5	1.1	0.0	146
Light (350ml)	4.6	0.0	4.6	0.7	0.0	99
Lager (100ml)	Trace	Trace	Trace	0.3	Trace	29
Lager, low-alcohol (100ml)	1.5	Trace	1.5	0.2	0	10
Lager, alcohol-free (100ml)	1.5	Trace	1.5	0.4	Trace	7
Lager, premium (100ml)	2.4	Trace	2.4	0.3	Trace	59
COCKTAILS						
Bloody Mary (100ml)	3.3	0.3	3.0	0.5	0.1	77
Margarita (100ml)	13.9	0.1	13.8	0.1	0.1	219
Pina Colada (100ml)	24.9	0.4	24.5	0.5	2.1	191
Screwdriver (100ml)	8.6	0.2	8.5	0.5	0.1	85
SHERRY, DRY (100ml)	1.4	0.0	1.4	0.2	0	72
SPIRITS (whisky, gin, rum, vodka, etc., any proof) (25ml)	0.0	0.0	0.0	0.0	0	82

Food Item (Amount)	Carb (g)	Fibre (g)	Net Carbs (g)	Protein (g)	Fat (g)	Cals
WINE						
Dessert, dry (100ml)	4.2	0.0	4.2	0.2	0	130
Dessert, sweet (100ml)	12.2	0.0	12.2	0.2	0	158
Non-alcoholic (100ml)	1.1	0.0	1.1	0.5	0	6
Red (100ml)	1.8	0.0	1.8	0.2	0	74
White (100ml)	0.8	0.0	0.8	0.1	0	70

BREADS, BUNS AND CRACKERS

It is important to be able to judge portions by eye when it comes to breads, muffins and bagels because unit size varies greatly (see pages 21–2). A deli bagel or muffin can easily pack a day's worth of carbs. The best choices are controlled carbohydrate baked goods. When they aren't available, opt for multigrain or wholewheat breads in slices about the size of your palm. Before eating crackers or breadsticks, separate the number you want to eat, then put the package away. When you've finished your allotment, don't reach for more. (This is a good way to prevent mindless munching.) Toast bread whenever possible – crunchy food takes longer to chew. And once you're in the Lifetime Maintenance phase and choose to eat conventional bread, opt for open sandwiches instead of standard ones.

Food Item (Amount)	Carb (g)	Fibre (g)	Net Carbs (g)	Protein (g)	Fat (g)	Cals
Bagel						
Cinnamon Raisin (11cm)	65.1	2.7	62.4	11.6	2.0	323
Plain (9cm)	37.9	1.6	36.3	7.5	1.1	195
Plain, poppy, sesame (11cm)	58.7	2.5	56.2	11.6	1.8	303
Bread						
BREADSTICK						
Sesame (1 small)	2.0	0.0	2.0	0.0	0.0	15
Brown bread (100g)	42.1	3.5	38.6	7.9	2.0	207
Chapatis (100g)	48.3	not known	not known	8.1	12.8	328
Ciabatta (100g)	52.0	2.3	49.7	10.2	3.9	271
Fruit malt loaf (100g)	64.9	2.6	62.3	7.8	2.3	295
Granary (100g)	47.4	3.3	44.1	9.6	2.3	237
Italian (25g slice)	14.2	0.8	13.4	2.5	1.0	77
Naan (100g)	50.2	2.0	48.2	7.8	7.3	285
Pitta, white (17cm diameter)	33.4	1.3	32.1	5.5	0.7	165
Pitta, wholewheat (17cm diameter)	35.2	4.7	30.5	6.3	1.7	170
Pumpernickel (25g slice)	13.5	1.8	11.6	2.5	0.9	71
Raisin (25g slice)	14.8	1.2	13.6	2.2	1.3	78
Rye (25g slice)	13.7	1.6	12.1	2.4	0.9	73
Sourdough (25g slice)	14.7	0.9	13.9	2.5	0.9	78
Wheat (25g slice)	13.4	1.2	12.2	2.6	1.2	74
White (25g slice)	14.0	0.7	13.4	2.3	1.0	76
WHITE SLICED (100G)						
Danish-style	44.5	2.4	42.1	9.1	2.7	228
Farmhouse	48.4	2.1	46.3	9.0	2.0	236
French stick	56.1	2.4	53.7	9.0	1.9	263
Mighty White with added fibre	49.6	3.1	46.5	7.6	1.5	230

Food Item (Amount)	Carb (g)	Fibre (g)	Net Carbs (g)	Protein (g)	Fat (g)	Cals
Premium	47.0	1.9	45.1	8.3	2.3	230
Whole grain (25g slice)	13.4	1.2	12.2	2.6	1.2	74
Wholemeal (100g)	42.0	5.0	37	9.4	2.5	217
Buns (100g)						
Chelsea buns	55.8	1.7	54.1	7.8	14.2	368
Crumpets	45.4	0	45.4	6.9	1.0	207
Currant buns	52.6	2.2	50.4	8.0	5.6	280
Custard tarts (1)	32.4	1.2	31.2	6.3	14.5	277
Eccles cakes	56.3	1.5	54.8	4.0	17.8	387
Hot cross buns	58.4	1.9	56.5	7.4	7.0	312
Muffins, English	44.2	1.9	42.3	10	1.9	223
SCONES						
Fruit	56.2	2.0	54.2	6.5	8.7	315
Plain	53.7	1.9	51.8	7.2	14.8	364
Wholemeal	43.0	5.2	37.8	8.8	14.6	328
Scotch pancakes	43.0	1.5	41.5	5.6	9.6	270
Crackers						
100% Stoned Wheat (3)	8.2	1.2	7.0	1.1	2.1	53
Brown rice snaps (8)	11.0	1.0	10.0	1.0	0.0	50
Cream crackers (100g)	68.3	2.2	66.1	9.5	13.3	414
Crispbread, rye (100g)	70.6	11.7	58.9	9.4	0.6	308
Melba toast (2)	7.7	0.6	7.1	1.2	0.3	39
Ritz (5)	10.0	0.0	10.0	1.0	4.0	80
Water biscuits (100g)	75.8	3.1	72.7	10.8	12.5	440
Water biscuits, Carr's (5)	13.0	1.0	12.0	2.0	1.5	70
Wheat thins (8)	10.0	0.4	9.6	1.2	5.9	68
Wholemeal crackers (100g)	72.0	4.4	67.6	10.1	11.5	414

Food Item (Amount)	Carb (g)	Fibre (g)	Net Carbs (g)	Protein (g)	Fat (g)	Cals
Muffin (50g)						
Banana nut (1)	29.0	1.0	28.0	3.0	7.0	190
Blueberry (1)	27.2	1.5	25.8	3.1	3.7	157
Bran (1)	23.7	4.0	19.7	4.0	7.3	163
Corn (1)	28.9	1.9	26.9	3.4	4.8	173
Roll						
Dinner (25g)	14.3	0.9	13.4	2.4	2.1	85
Hamburger (40g)	21.7	1.3	20.4	3.6	3.1	129
White, hard (25g)	14.9	0.7	14.3	2.8	1.2	83
Whole wheat (25g)	14.5	2.1	12.4	2.5	1.3	75
Scone						
Homemade (7cm)	26.8	0.9	25.9	4.2	9.8	212
Tortillas						
Corn (1)	12.1	1.4	10.7	1.5	0.6	58
Flour (1)	27.2	1.6	25.6	4.3	3.5	159
Wholewheat (1)	20.0	1.9	18.1	2.9	0.4	73

CEREALS AND CEREAL BARS

Fibre counts here, because it accounts for the major differences in grams of Net Carbs. Therefore, when you are on Pre-Maintenance and Lifetime Maintenance, opt for fibre-rich whole grain products with no added sugar. (The less said about multi-coloured puffed cereal coated with sugar, the better!) The counts given are for 2-tablespoon servings: not very big amounts for a lot of carbs – so add cereals only when you are near your goal weight. A better option is to only eat controlled carb products. Most cereal bars contain sugar, and should be avoided.

Food Item (Amount)	Carb (g)	Fibre (g)	Net Carbs (g)	Protein (g)	Fat (g)	Cals
Cereals (100g)						
Cheerios	74.6	6.5	68.1	8.1	3.9	366
Jordans organic crunch	66.3	6.4	59.9	8.1	13.5	not known
KELLOGGS						
Bran flakes	66	15	51	10	2.5	330
Cornflakes	84	2.5	81.5	7.0	0.8	370
Crunchy nut cornflakes	83	2.5	80.5	6.0	3.5	390
Fruit 'n' fibre	71	9.0	62	8.0	5.0	360
Special K	75	2.5	72.5	16.0	1.0	370
Sultana Bran	66	13	53	8.0	2.5	320
Muesli	62.3	9.3	53	9.9	10.2	not known
Porridge oats, Scott's	61.5	8.0	53.5	12.5	7.4	368

Food Item (Amount)	Carb (g)	Fibre (g)	Net Carbs (g)	Protein (g)	Fat (g)	Cals
Rice Krispies	87	1.0	86	6.0	1.0	380
Shreddies	71.7	11.2	60.5	9.8	1.9	not known
Sporties	77.2	8.5	68.7	8.5	1.6	not known
Sugar puffs	86.5	3.0	83.5	6.5	1.0	387
Shredded wheat	66.1	11.5	54.6	11.2	2.1	330
Breakfast bars						
Alpen, original	26.4	3.1	23.3	4.0	2.7	
Alpen, no added sugar	24.5	3.6	20.9	4.8	2.8	
Cornflakes cereal bar	18	0.4	17.6	2.5	4.5	
Jordans muesli break	30.6	2.0	28.6	2.7	5.0	
Nutri-grain, apple	26	1.0	25	1.5	3.5	
Nutri-grain, strawberry	26	1.0	25	1.5	3.5	
Nutri-grain, chocolate	23	1.5	21.5	1.5	4.0	
Porridge oats bar	62	7.0	55	11	0.8	
Rice Krispies cereal bar	13	0.1	12.9	2.0	3.5	
Special K bar	18	0.2	17.8	1.5	1.5	

BREAKFAST PASTRIES

Commercial breakfast pastries – even those weighing a scant 50g – are made with white flour, sugar and sweet fillings – and all are loaded with carbs. The best advice we can give you is to stay away from them.

Food Item (Amount)	Carb (g)	Fibre (g)	Net Carbs (g)	Protein (g)	Fat (g)	Cals
Breakfast Pastries						
Bagels (100g)	57.8	2.4	55.4	10.0	1.8	273
Croissants (100g)	43.3	1.6	41.7	8.3	19.7	373
DANISH						
Plain (100g)	51.3	1.6	49.7	5.8	14.1	342
Cinnamon (50g)	25.3	0.7	24.6	4.0	12.7	229
Entenmann's, Pecan Pastry						
Ring (50g)	24.6	1.1	23.5	3.2	16.1	246
Eclairs, Frozen (Bird's Eye)	26.1	0.8	25.3	5.6	30.6	396
FRENCH TOAST						
Homemade (50g piece)	16.3	0.6	15.7	5.0	7.0	149
Pancakes						
Plain (100g)	34.9	0.8	34.1	6.0	16.3	302
Scotch pancakes (see p. 31)						
Toaster Pastry						
Frosted Pop Tart (1)	37.4	0.5	36.9	2.2	5.3	204
Pop Tart (1)	32.2	0.8	31.5	2.7	9.2	219

Scotch pancakes (see p. 31)

FRUIT

Berries are the preferred fruit on Atkins, because of their high fibre content and relatively low carb count. Keep portion size in mind, though, because a small handful of berries – the recommended quantity – is a small amount. One trick to make berries last longer is to pop them in the freezer and eat them partially frozen. Kiwi fruit is another good option; it's loaded with vitamins and contains only 8.7g of Net Carbs per fruit. Rhubarb, which needs to be cooked, is an often overlooked choice. It is excellent when prepared with sugar substitute and lemon peel. Dried fruits, such as raisins, prunes and dates are much higher in carbs than their fresh counterparts. Keep in mind that whole fruit is always a better choice than fruit juice, which is higher in carbs and missing all or much of the fibre.

Food Item (Amount)	Carb (g)	Fibre (g)	Net Carbs (g)	Protein (g)	Fat (g)	Cals
Apple (½ medium)	10.5	1.9	8.7	0.1	0.3	41
APPLESAUCE						
Sweetened (2tbs)	25.4	1.5	23.9	0.2	0.2	97
Unsweetened (2tbs)	13.8	1.5	12.3	0.2	0.1	52
APRICOTS						
Tinned, in juice (3 halves)	13.3	1.7	11.6	0.7	0.0	52
Dried, (6 halves)	13.0	1.9	11.1	0.8	0.1	50
Fresh (3 whole)	11.7	2.5	9.2	1.5	0.4	50
AVOCADO						
California (Haas) (½)	6.0	4.2	1.7	1.8	15.0	153
Florida (½)	13.5	8.1	5.5	2.4	13.5	170
Banana, small (1)	23.7	2.4	21.2	1.0	0.5	93
Banana chips (1tbs)	13.4	1.8	11.7	0.5	7.7	119
BLACKBERRIES						
Fresh (2tbs)	9.2	3.8	5.4	0.5	0.3	37
Frozen, unsweetened (2tbs)	11.8	3.8	8.1	0.9	0.3	48
BLUEBERRIES						
Fresh (2tbs)	10.2	2.0	8.3	0.5	0.3	41
Frozen, sweetened (2tbs)	25.2	2.4	22.8	0.5	0.2	93
Frozen, unsweetened (2tbs)	9.4	2.1	7.4	0.3	0.5	40
BOYSENBERRIES						
Fresh (2tbs)	9.2	3.8	5.4	0:5	0.3	37
Frozen, unsweetened (2tbs)	8.1	2.6	5.5	0.7	0.2	33
Cherimoya (2tbs)	27.0	2.7	24.3	1.5	0.5	106
Cranberries, raw, no sugar (2tbs)	6.0	2.0	4.0	0.2	0.1	23

Food Item (Amount)	Carb (g)	Fibre (g)	Net Carbs (g)	Protein (g)	Fat (g)	Cals
DATES						
Chopped (2tbs)	65.4	6.7	58.8	1.8	0.4	245
Fresh (3)	18.3	1.9	16.4	0.5	0.1	68
FIGS						
Tinned, in water (2tbs)	17.4	2.7	14.6	0.5	0.1	66
Fresh, small (1)	7.7	1.3	6.4	0.3	0.1	30
FRUIT COCKTAIL						
Tinned, in heavy syrup (2tbs)	23.5	1.2	22.2	0.5	0.1	91
Tinned, in water (2tbs)	10.1	1.2	8.9	0.5	0.1	38
FRUIT SALAD						
Tinned, in heavy syrup (2tbs)	24.4	1.3	23.1	0.4	0.1	93
Tinned, in juice (2tbs)	16.3	1.3	15.0	0.6	0.0	62
Gooseberries, raw, no sugar (2tbs)	7.6	3.2	4.4	0.7	0.4	33
GRAPEFRUIT						
Fresh (2tbs)	9.5	1.7	7.8	0.7	0.1	37
Sections (2tbs)	9.3	1.3	8.0	0.7	0.1	37
GRAPES						
Green seedless (2tbs)	14.2	0.8	13.4	0.5	0.5	57
Black (2tbs)	7.9	0.5	7.4	0.3	0.2	31
Guava (2tbs)	9.8	4.5	5.3	0.7	0.5	42
Guava paste (2tbs)	20.6	0.3	20.3	0.0	0.0	80
JUICES (see Beverages – non-alcoholic)						
Kiwifruit (1)	11.3	2.6	8.7	0.8	0.3	46
Kumquat (4)	12.5	5.0	7.5	0.7	0.1	48
Lemon juice (2tbs)	2.6	0.1	2.5	0.1	0.0	8
Loganberries (2tbs)	9.2	3.8	5.4	0.5	0.3	37

Food Item (Amount)	Carb (g)	Fibre (g)	Net Carbs (g)	Protein (g)	Fat (g)	Cals
Loquat, small (10)	16.5	2.3	14.2	0.6	0.3	64
LYCHEES						
Fresh (2tbs)	15.7	1.2	14.5	0.8	0.4	63
Fresh, whole (10)	15.9	1.3	14.6	0.8	0.4	63
MANGO						
Dried (1 piece)	8.0	0.0	8.0	0.0	0.3	33
Fresh (2tbs)	14.0	1.5	12.5	0.4	0.2	54
MELON						
Cantaloupe						
Balls (2tbs)	7.4	0.7	6.7	0.8	0.3	31
Medium (13cm diameter, 1/2)	23.1	2.2	20.9	2.4	0.8	97
Honeydew, balls (2tbs)	7.8	0.5	7.3	0.4	0.1	30
Watermelon, balls (2tbs)	5.5	0.4	5.1	0.5	0.3	25
Nectarine (1)	16.0	2.2	13.8	1.3	0.6	67
ORANGE						
Sections (2tbs)	10.6	2.2	8.4	0.9	0.1	42
Whole (1)	16.3	3.4	12.9	1.4	0.1	64
PAPAYA						
Dried (1 piece)	14.9	2.7	12.2	0.9	0.2	59
Fresh, small 1/2	7.5	1.4	6.1	0.5	0.1	30
Passion Fruit (1tbs)	13.8	6.1	7.7	1.3	0.4	57
PEACH						
Tinned, in water (2tbs)	7.5	1.6	5.9	0.5	0.1	29
Dried, halves (2)	16.0	2.1	13.8	0.9	0.2	62
Fresh, small (1)	8.8	1.6	7.2	0.6	0.1	34
PEAR						
Tinned, in juice (100g)	8.5	1.4	7.1	0.3	Trace	33
Tinned, in syrup (100g)	13.2	1.1	12.1	0.2	Trace	50

Food Item (Amount)	Carb (g)	Fibre (g)	Net Carbs (g)	Protein (g)	Fat (g)	Cals
Tinned, in water, halves (2tbs)	9.5	2.0	7.6	0.2	0.0	35
Fresh, medium, Bartlett (1)	25.1	4.0	21.1	0.7	0.7	98
Fresh, small, Bosc (1)	21.0	3.3	17.7	0.5	0.6	82
Persimmon, large (1/2)	15.6	3.0	12.6	0.5	0.2	59
PINEAPPLE						
Tinned, in juice (100g)	12.2	0.5	11.7	0.3	Trace	47
Tinned, in syrup (100g)	16.5	0.7	15.8	0.5	Trace	64
Tinned, in water (2tbs)	10.2	1.0	9.2	0.5	0.1	39
Fresh, chunks (2tbs)	9.6	0.9	8.7	0.3	0.3	38
PLUM						
Dried (prune) (4)	21.1	2.4	18.7	0.9	0.2	80
Dried (prune), tinned, in heavy syrup (2tbs)	32.5	4.5	28.1	1.0	0.2	123
Fresh, small (1)	3.7	0.4	3.3	0.2	0.2	16
Purple, tinned, in water (2tbs)	13.7	1.3	12.5	0.5	0.0	51
Pomegranate (1/4)	6.6	0.2	6.4	0.4	0.1	26
PRUNES						
Tinned, in juice (100g)	19.7	2.4	14.3	0.7	0.2	79
Tinned, in syrup (100g)	23.0	2.8	20.2	0.6	0.2	90
Ready to eat (100g)	34.0	5.7	28.3	2.5	0.4	141
RAISINS						
Seedless (1tbs)	8.1	0.7	7.4	0.3	0.1	31
Sultanas (1tbs)	8.2	0.4	7.8	0.4	0.0	31
RASPBERRIES						
Tinned, in syrup (100g)	22.5	1.5	21.0	0.6	0.1	88
Fresh (2tbs)	7.1	4.2	3.0	0.6	0.3	30

Food Item (Amount)	Carb (g)	Fibre (g)	Net Carbs (g)	Protein (g)	Fat (g)	Cals
Frozen, sweetened (2tbs)	32.7	5.5	27.2	0.9	0.2	129
RHUBARB						
Tinned, in syrup (100g)	7.6	0.8	6.8	0.5	Trace	31
Fresh (2tbs)	2.8	1.1	1.7	0.6	0.1	13
Stewed, with sugar (100g)	11.5	1.2	10.3	0.9	0.1	48
STRAWBERRIES						
Tinned, in syrup (100g)	16.9	0.7	16.2	0.5	Trace	65
Fresh, whole (2tbs)	5.1	1.7	3.4	0.4	0.3	22
Frozen, sweetened (2tbs)	33.0	2.4	30.6	0.7	0.2	122
Frozen, unsweetened (2tbs)	6.8	1.6	5.2	0.3	0.1	26
Tangerine, small (1)	7.8	1.6	6.2	0.4	0.1	31

EGGS AND CHEESE

Most hard cheeses are full fat, low in carbs and can be enjoyed on all phases of Atkins. You can eat fresh cheeses, such as ricotta and cottage cheese, after Induction. Be wary of 'cheese products' and 'cheese spreads' because they are higher in carbs and often highly processed. Serving size counts here: cheese is a dense food. 25g of hard cheese is really small – about the size of a pair of dice. Add volume to cheese by grating it.

Food Item (Amount)	Carb (g)	Fibre (g)	Net Carbs (g)	Protein (g)	Fat (g)	Cals
Eggs						
Fried (1)	0.6	0.0	0.6	6.2	6.9	92
Poached/boiled (1)	0.6	0.0	0.6	6.3	5.3	78
Quiche Lorraine (100g)	19.6	0.7	18.9	13.7	25.5	358
Quiche, cheese + egg	17.1	0.6	16.5	12.4	22.3	315
Quiche, cheese + egg, wholemeal	14.3	1.8	12.5	13.1	22.5	309
Scrambled, with milk (1)	1.3	0.0	1.3	6.8	7.5	101
Scrambled, egg substitute (2tbs)	1.4	0.0	1.4	3.6	4.1	58
White, uncooked (50ml)	0.6	0.0	0.6	6.0	0.0	29
Cheese						
Blue, crumbled (25g)	0.4	0.0	0.4	3.6	4.9	60
Boursin (25g)	1.0	0.0	1.0	2.0	13.0	120

Food Item (Amount)	Carb (g)	Fibre (g)	Net Carbs (g)	Protein (g)	Fat (g)	Cals
Brie (25g)	0.1	0.0	0.1	5.9	7.9	95
Camembert (25g)	0.1	0.0	0.1	5.6	6.9	85
Cheddar (25g)	0.4	0.0	0.4	7.1	9.4	114
Cottage, 2% fat (100g)	4.1	0.0	4.1	15.5	2.2	101
Cottage, creamed (100g)	2.8	0.0	2.8	13.1	4.7	109
Cracker Barrel (25g)	4.0	0.0	4.0	5.0	8.0	100
CREAM						
Chive & Onion (25g)	2.0	0.0	2.0	2.0	10.0	110
Plain (25g)	0.8	0.0	0.8	2.2	10.1	101
Edam (25g)	0.4	0.0	0.4	7.1	7.9	101
Feta (25g)	1.2	0.0	1.2	4.0	6.0	75
Fontina (25g)	0.4	0.0	0.4	7.3	8.8	110
Goat, soft (25g)	0.3	0.0	0.3	5.3	6.0	76
Gorgonzola (25g)	0.0	0.0	0.0	7.0	9.0	111
Gouda (25g)	0.6	0.0	0.6	7.1	7.8	101
Havarti (25g)	0.8	0.0	0.8	6.6	8.4	105
Jarlsberg (25g)	1.0	0.0	1.0	8.1	7.8	107
Laughing Cow (1 wedge)	1.0	0.0	1.0	2.0	4.0	50
Mascarpone (25g)	0.6	0.0	0.6	2.0	13.2	126
Mozzarella, whole milk (25g)	0.6	0.0	0.6	5.5	6.1	80
Mozzarella, part skim (25g)	0.8	0.0	0.8	6.9	4.5	72
Muenster (25g)	0.3	0.0	0.3	6.6	8.5	104
Neuchatel (25g)	2.0	0.0	2.0	3.0	5.0	70
Parmesan, chunk (25g)	0.9	0.0	0.9	10.1	7.3	111
Parmesan, grated (15g)	0.2	0.0	0.2	2.6	1.9	28
Processed (1 slice, 8g)	0.3	0.0	0.3	4.7	6.6	79
Provolone (25g)	0.6	0.0	0.6	7.3	7.6	100
Ricotta, whole milk (100g)	1.9	0.0	1.9	6.9	8.0	107

Food Item (Amount)	Carb (g)	Fibre (g)	Net Carbs (g)	Protein (g)	Fat (g)	Cals
Ricotta, part skim (100g)	3.2	0.0	3.2	7.0	4.9	85
Romano, chunk (25g)	1.0	0.0	1.0	9.1	7.1	105
Romano, grated (15g)	0.2	0.0	0.2	2.0	1.7	24
Swiss (25g)	1.0	0.0	1.0	8.1	7.8	107

MILK, CREAM, BUTTER AND YOGURT

Most low-fat yogurts (and there are a zillion of them) are high in carbohydrates. For a much lower-carb – and better-tasting – fruit yogurt, buy whole milk yogurt, sweeten it with sugar substitute and mix in chopped berries. As for sour cream and double cream, note that the carb count given is for small amounts (2 tablespoons and 1 tablespoon respectively), so keep that in mind when topping vegetables or adding cream to your decaf coffee.

Food Item (Amount)	Carb (g)	Fibre (g)	Net Carbs (g)	Protein (g)	Fat (g)	Cals
Butter						
Butter (15g)	0.0	0.0	0.0	0.1	11.5	102
Butter, spreadable (15g)	0.0	0.0	0.0	0.0	7.0	70
Cream						
Double, liquid (1tbs)	0.4	0.0	0.4	0.3	5.5	51
Double, whipped (2tbs)	0.4	0.0	0.4	0.3	5.5	52
Single (1tbs)	0.6	0.0	0.6	0.4	2.9	29
Clotted cream (100g)	2.2	0.0	2.2	0.0	63.5	587
CREAMER, NON-DAIRY						
Coffeemate Plain (1tbs)	2.0	0.0	2.0	0.0	1.0	20
Milk						
BUTTERMILK						
Cultured from 1% milk (250ml)	13.0	0.0	13.0	9.0	2.5	110

Food Item (Amount)	Carb (g)	Fibre (g)	Net Carbs (g)	Protein (g)	Fat (g)	Cals
Cultured from skimmed milk (250ml)	11.7	0.0	11.7	8.1	2.2	99
Condensed, tinned (2tbs)	20.8	0.0	20.8	3.0	3.3	123
Evaporated, 2% fat (2tbs)	3.5	0.0	3.5	2.3	0.6	29
Evaporated, whole (2tbs)	3.2	0.0	3.2	2.2	2.4	42
Lowfat (1%) (250ml)	11.7	0.0	11.7	8.0	2.6	102
Non-fat (skimmed) (250ml)	11.9	0.0	11.9	8.4	0.4	86
Reduced fat, 2% (250ml)	11.7	0.0	11.7	8.1	4.7	121
Whole (250ml)	11.4	0.0	11.4	8.0	8.2	150
FLAVOURED MILK						
(See Beverages, non-alcoholic)						
RICE MILK						
Plain (250ml)	25.0	0.0	25.0	1.0	2.0	120
Vanilla (250ml)	28.0	0.0	28.0	1.0	2.0	130
SOYA MILK						
Plain (250ml)	4.4	3.2	1.2	6.7	4.7	81
Sour Cream						
Regular (2tbs)	1.2	0.0	1.2	0.9	6.0	62
Yogurt						
DANONE ACTIVA (125g)						
Natural	7.5	0	7.5	5.4	4.3	90
Peach	11.1	0	11.1	4.6	0.1	64
Raspberry	16	0	16	4.5	3.5	113
MULLER LIGHT (100g)						
Chocolate	8.1	0	8.1	4.8	0.3	54
Raspberry and cream	8.3	0	8.3	4.4	0.1	52
Toffee	8.5	0	8.5	4.4	0.1	53
Vanilla	8.3	0	8.3	4.6	0.1	53

Food Item (Amount)	Carb (g)	Fibre (g)	Net Carbs (g)	Protein (g)	Fat (g)	Cals
MULLER VITALITY PROBIOTIC (100g)						
Raspberry	15.4	0	15.4	4.8	1.8	97
Strawberry	15.6	0	15.6	4.7	1.8	97
PLAIN						
Lowfat (225g)	15.0	0.0	15.0	11.0	3.0	130
Whole milk (250ml)	11.0	0.0	11.0	9.0	8.0	150
SKI LOW FAT (125g)						
Peach	20.4	0	20.4	6.1	2.4	128
Strawberry	19.8	0	19.8	6	2.3	124
Vanilla	19.6	0	19.6	6.1	2.3	124
ST IVEL SHAPE (120g)						
Simply berries	6.7	0.3	6.4	5.5	0.2	53
TOTAL GREEK (100g)						
Plain	4	0	4	6	10	130
YEO VALLEY (100g)						
Cranberry and apple	13.1	0.2	12.9	5.1	0.1	74
Natural	6.6	0	6.6	4.5	4.2	82
Strawberry and wholegrain	13.1	0.1	13	4.0	3.8	103
YOPLAIT						
Custard (175g)	32.0	0.0	32.0	7.0	3.5	190
Expresse (1)	11.0	0.0	11.0	2.0	1.5	70
Light (175g)	19.0	0.0	19.0	5-6	0.0	100
Original (175g)	33.0	0.0	33.0	5	1.5	170

SWEETENERS, JAMS AND SYRUPS

Unsweetened jams and preserves are naturally sweet and, when portions are small, are low in carbohydrates. Other good choices include products sweetened with sucralose (Splenda). It is always important to pay attention to serving size. A good rule of thumb is that one teaspoon of jam will thinly cover a slice of bread. Also note that packets of sugar substitute each contain about 1g of carbohydrate, so if you sweeten six cups of herbal tea in one day, the carbs can add up.

Food Item (Amount)	Carb (g)	Fibre (g)	Net Carbs (g)	Protein (g)	Fat (g)	Cals
Jam/Preserves/Spreads						
Chocolate nut spread (100g)	60.5	0.8	59.7	6.2	33.0	549
Jam/preserves (1tsp)	4.6	0.1	4.5	0.0	0.0	19
Lemon curd (100g)	62.7	0.2	62.5	0.6	4.9	282
Marmalade (100g)	69.5	0.3	69.2	0.1	0	261
Marmite (100g)	0.8	0.1	0.7	1.5	0	9
Peanut butter (100g)	22.4	5.9	16.5	22.2	53	590
Reduced sugar (1tsp)	3.0	0.2	2.8	0.1	0.1	12
Syrups						
Golden Syrup (1tbs)	15.7	0.0	15.7	0.0	0.0	58
Honey (1tsp)	5.8	0.0	5.8	0.0	0.0	21
Treacle (1tsp)	4.4	0.0	4.4	0.0	0.0	17

Food Item (Amount)	Carb (g)	Fibre (g)	Net Carbs (g)	Protein (g)	Fat (g)	Cals
Ice-cream sauce (topping, all flavours)	53.9	0	53.9	0.8	0.2	207
PANCAKE SYRUP						
Maple (1tbs)	13.4	0.0	13.4	0.0	0.0	52
Maple-flavoured (1tbs)	15.1	0.0	15.1	0.0	0.0	57
Reduced calorie (1tbs)	6.6	0.0	6.6	0.0	0.0	25
Sugar						
Brown, packed (1tsp)	4.5	0.0	4.5	0.0	0.0	17
Demerara sugar (100g)	104.5	0	104.5	0.5	0	394
Granulated sugar (100g)	105.0	0	105.0	Trace	0	394
Powdered, unsifted (1tsp)	2.5	0.0	2.5	0.0	0.0	10
White (1tsp)	4.2	0.0	4.2	0.0	0.0	16
Sweeteners						
Canderel (1tsp)	0.47	0.0	0.47	0.01	0.0	1.9
Hermesetas (1tsp)	0.28	0.21	0.28	0.01	0.0	1.4
Sweetex (100g)	0.0	0.0	0.0	0.0	Trace	Trace
Sweet'N Low (1 packet)	1.0	0.0	1.0	0.0	0.0	0

SAUCES, GRAVIES, MARINADES AND DIPS

Reading labels is extremely important in this category. Not only do carb counts vary widely, but many sauces also contain corn syrups and hydrogenated oils, which should be avoided. Be especially careful when buying tomato sauce: find a brand low in carbs that you like and stock up on it. Marinades are minimally absorbed by the foods they coat, so you may safely halve the total carb count given for marinades. But do avoid slathering barbecue sauce on grilled food – not only will it burn, but more doesn't mean tastier and only adds extra carbs.

Food Item (Amount)	Carb (g)	Fibre (g)	Net Carbs (g)	Protein (g)	Fat (g)	Cals
Sauces						
Barbecue sauce (100g)	23.4	0.5	22.9	1.0	0.1	93
Bread sauce (100g)	15.2	0.6	14.6	4.1	4.0	110
Brown sauce (100g)	22.2	0.7	21.5	1.2	0.1	98
Cheese sauce (100g)	8.7	0.2	8.5	8.1	14.8	198
CHUTNEY						
Apple	49.2	1.3	47.9	0.9	0.2	190
Mango	49.5	0.9	48.6	0.4	10.9	285
Tomato	31.0	1.3	29.7	1.2	0.2	128
Cranberry Sauce, whole or jellied (2tbs)	13.0	0.5	12.5	0.0	0.0	50

Food Item (Amount)	Carb (g)	Fibre (g)	Net Carbs (g)	Protein (g)	Fat (g)	Cals
Hollandaise sauce (2tbs)	1.7	0.1	1.6	0.6	2.5	30
Onion sauce (100g)	8.1	0.4	7.7	2.9	6.6	101
Peanut sauce (2tbs)	3.6	0.9	2.7	3.9	7.9	94
Pesto sauce (2tbs)	2.0	0.9	1.2	5.6	14.2	155
TACO SAUCE						
Green (1tbs)	0.9	0.1	0.8	0.1	0.0	5
Red, (1tbs)	1.0	0.0	1.0	0.0	0.0	5
Tartare sauce	17.9	Trace	17.9	1.3	24.6	299
Soy Sauce	8.2	0.0	8.2	3.0	Trace	43
TOMATO SAUCE						
Tinned (2tbs)	4.4	0.9	3.5	0.8	0.1	18
Tomato Ketchup (100g)	28.6	0.9	27.7	1.6	0.1	115
Tomato Purée (100g)	14.2	2.8	11.4	5.0	0.3	76
White sauce (100g)	10.6	0.2	10.4	4.2	10.3	151
White (sweet) sauce (100g)	18.3	0.2	18.1	3.9	9.5	171
Gravy						
Beef (2tbs)	1.4	0.1	1.3	1.1	0.7	15
Chicken (2tbs)	1.6	0.1	1.5	0.6	1.7	24
Turkey (2tbs)	1.5	0.1	1.4	0.8	0.6	15
Dips						
Cheese and chive (100g)	2.7	0.7	2.0	3.9	40.4	390
Hummus (100g)	8.9	2.2	6.7	7.3	27.5	312
Onion and garlic (100g)	4.8	0.9	3.9	1.5	63.1	593
Sour cream and chive (100g)	2.5	0.1	2.4	2.2	2.8	316
Taramasalata (100g)	7.5	0.1	7.4	4.0	48.1	479

Food Item (Amount)	Carb (g)	Fibre (g)	Net Carbs (g)	Protein (g)	Fat (g)	Cals
Marinades						
Cardini's Zesty Lemon Pepper (100g)	22	0.6	22	0.3	0.3	90
SAINSBURY						
Date & Harissa						
North African (100g)	15.7	3.2	15.7	1.2	14.0	194
Sticky barbecue (100g)	24.3	0.4	24.3	0.7	0.3	104
Salsa						
Doritos (2tbs)	3.0	1.0	2.0	1.0	0.0	15
Green (2tbs)	1.0	0.0	1.0	0.0	0.0	10
Red (2tbs)	2.0	0.5	1.5	0.4	0.1	9

SEASONINGS AND CONDIMENTS

These products add flavour to most other foods, so keep a variety in your pantry and refrigerator. With the exception of commercial ketchup (which contains corn syrup), most are low in carbs because their intense flavours mean you only need to consume small amounts. A quick tip: to make your own sweet relish, chop up dill pickles, sprinkle with sugar substitute and marinate in the refrigerator for a day.

Food Item (Amount)	Carb (g)	Fibre (g)	Net Carbs (g)	Protein (g)	Fat (g)	Cals
Anchovies, in oil, drained (1)	0.0	0.0	0.0	1.2	0.4	8
Basil, fresh (1tbs)	0.1	0.1	0.0	0.1	0.0	1
Capers (1tbs)	0.4	0.3	0.1	0.2	0.1	2
Caponata (2tbs)	2.0	2.0	0.0	0.0	2.0	25
Chili powder (1tsp)	1.4	0.9	0.5	0.3	0.4	8
Chives (1tbs)	0.1	0.1	0.1	0.1	0.0	1
Coriander, fresh (1tbs)	0.1	0.1	0.0	0.1	0.0	1
Cumin seed (1tsp)	0.9	0.2	0.7	0.4	0.5	7
Dill, fresh (1tbs)	0.0	0.0	0.0	0.0	0.0	0
Fish sauce (1tsp)	0.2	0.0	0.2	0.3	0.0	2
Garlic, clove (1)	1.0	0.1	0.9	0.2	0.0	4
Ginger root (1tbs)	0.9	0.1	0.8	0.1	0.0	4
Herbs, dried (oregano, thyme, etc) (1tsp)	1.0	0.6	0.4	0.2	0.2	5

Food Item (Amount)	Carb (g)	Fibre (g)	Net Carbs (g)	Protein (g)	Fat (g)	Cals
Hoisin sauce (2tbs)	2.0	1.0	1.0	0.0	0.0	15
Horseradish, prepared (1tsp)	0.6	0.2	0.4	0.1	0.0	2
Ketchup (100g)	28.6	0.9	27.7	1.6	0.1	115
Miso paste (1tbs)	3.0	0.4	2.6	1.9	0.8	27
Mustard, Dijon (1tsp)	0.6	0.1	0.5	0.3	0.5	
Mustard, yellow (1tsp)	0.4	0.2	0.2	0.2	0.2	3
Olives, black, large (5)	1.4	0.7	0.7	0.2	2.4	25
Olives, green (5)	0.3	0.2	0.1	0.3	2.5	23
Parsley, fresh (1tbs)	0.2	0.1	0.1	0.1	0.0	1
PEPPERS						
Hot cherry (1)	2.0	1.0	1.0	0.0	0.0	10
Hot red, tinned (1)	3.7	1.0	2.8	0.7	0.1	15
Jalapeño, pickled (1)	1.0	0.1	0.8	0.1	0.0	4
Roasted red (1)	1.5	0.0	1.5	0.0	0.0	5
Pickle, dill (1)	2.7	0.8	1.9	0.4	0.1	12
Pickle, relish (1tbs)	5.4	0.2	5.2	0.1	0.1	20
Pickle, sweet (1)	11.1	0.4	10.7	0.1	0.1	41
Sofrito (1tsp)	0.0	0.0	0.0	0.0	0.0	0
Soy sauce (1tbs)	1.5	0.0	1.5	0.9	0.0	10
Soy sauce, low sodium (1tbs)	1.4	0.1	1.2	0.8	0.0	8
Soy sauce, tamari (1tbs)	1.0	0.2	0.9	1.9	0.0	11
Steak sauce (1tbs)	2.4	0.3	2.1	0.2	0.0	9
Tabasco sauce (1tsp)	0.0	0.0	0.0	0.1	0.0	1
VINEGAR						
Balsamic (1tbs)	2.3	0.0	2.3	0.0	0.0	10
Cider (1tbs)	0.9	0.0	0.9	0.0	0.0	2
Red wine (1tbs)	1.5	0.0	1.5	0.0	0.0	5
Rice (1tbs)	0.0	0.0	0.0	0.0	0.0	0

Food Item (Amount)	Carb (g)	Fibre (g)	Net Carbs (g)	Protein (g)	Fat (g)	Cals
Rice, seasoned (1tbs)	3.0	0.0	3.0	0.0	0.0	12
White wine (1tbs)	0.0	0.0	0.0	0.0	0.0	5
Worcestershire Sauce (1tsp)	1.0	0.0	1.0	0.0	0.0	4

FATS, OILS AND SALAD DRESSINGS

A good dressing makes the salad, and fruity green olive oil will enhance just about any cooked vegetable. Enjoying healthful fats and oils is an important part of doing Atkins, and one of its pleasures. When you purchase commercial dressings, be sure to read the ingredient information on the label carefully: while most dressings are relatively low in carbs (except for sweet flavours, such as Honey Mustard), many do contain sugar, hydrogenated oils and artificial flavourings. Your local health food store is a good place to find brands with natural ingredients.

Food Item (Amount)	Carb (g)	Fibre (g)	Net Carbs (g)	Protein (g)	Fat (g)	Cals
Suet (100g)	12.1	0.5	11.6	Trace	86.7	826
Lard (1tbs)	0.0	0.0	0.0	0.0	12.8	116
Vegetable shortening (1tbs)	0.0	0.0	0.0	0.0	12.8	113
Oils, Salad and Cooking						
Corn (1tbs)	0.0	0.0	0.0	0.0	13.6	120
Olive (1tbs)	0.0	0.0	0.0	0.0	13.5	119
Peanut (1tbs)	0.0	0.0	0.0	0.0	13.5	119
Safflower (1tbs)	0.0	0.0	0.0	0.0	13.6	120
Sesame (1tbs)	0.0	0.0	0.0	0.0	13.6	120
Soya bean (1tbs)	0.0	0.0	0.0	0.0	13.6	120
Salad Dressing						
Blue cheese dressing (100g)	8.7	0	8.7	2.0	46.3	457

Food Item (Amount)	Carb (g)	Fibre (g)	Net Carbs (g)	Protein (g)	Fat (g)	Cals
French dressing (100g)	4.5	0	4.5	0.1	49.4	462
Kraft French dressing (2tbs)	4.0	0.0	4.0	0.0	12.0	120
Thousand Island dressing (100g)	12.5	0.4	12.1	1.1	30.2	323
Margarine / Butter						
Blended spread (Willow, Clover) (100g)	1.1	0	1.1	0.6	74.8	680
Butter (100g)	0.6	0	0.6	0.6	82.2	744
Flora Extra Light (100g)	1.8	0	1.8	4.9	37.6	365
Margarine, hard (1tbs)	0.1	0.0	0.1	0.1	11.4	101
Margarine, soft (1tbs)	0.1	0.0	0.1	0.1	11.4	102
Olivio (100g)	1.1	0.0	1.1	0.1	62.7	569
Outline low-fat spread (100g)	2.5	0	2.5	5.9	25.5	262
Mayonnaise						
Hellman's (1tbs)	0.1	0.0	0.1	0.2	11.2	100
Mayonnaise, plain (100g)	1.7	0	1.7	1.1	75.6	691
Mayonnaise, low-fat (100g)	8.2	0	8.2	1.0	28.1	288

SOUPS

The best soups are homemade. They are more flavourful and lower in sodium and carbohydrates – because you control the ingredients. Convenience counts though, and the smartest choices among prepared soups are vegetable soups, which are higher in fibre. Since most commercial soups pack at least 15 carb grams – and are only part of a meal – they should be included only when your metabolism allows for greater carbohydrate consumption. A good compromise in terms of convenience and nutritional value is adding fresh chopped cooked or raw veggies to reduced sodium broth. Crumble in a few reduced carb crackers for texture.

Food Item (Amount)	Carb (g)	Fibre (g)	Net Carbs (g)	Protein (g)	Fat (g)
BATCHELORS CUP A SOUP					
Chicken per serving	12.4	0.6	11.8	1.5	4.7
Oxtail	13.7	1	12.7	1.5	1.7
Golden vegetable	15.3	0.9	14.4	1	0.5
Rich tomato + basil	18.6	1.6	17	1.5	2.6
BAXTERS					
Tomato + orange ($^1/_2$ can)	17.5	1.0	16.5	2.3	1.0
Mulligatawny ($^1/_2$ can)	15.2	1.5	13.7	4.8	3.5
Chicken broth ($^1/_2$ can)	11.0	1.2	9.8	2.5	0.8
Spicy Parsnip ($^1/_2$ can)	12.7	3.1	9.6	2.3	5.2

Food Item (Amount)	Carb (g)	Fibre (g)	Net Carbs (g)	Protein (g)	Fat (g)	Cals
CAMPBELL'S CHUNKY						
Beef w/Country Vegetables (250ml)	18.0	3.0	15.0	13.0	4.0	160
Classic Chicken Noodle (250ml)	16.0	2.0	14.0	9.0	3.0	130
Minestrone (250ml)	22.0	2.0	20.0	5.0	5.0	140
Vegetable (250ml)	22.0	4.0	18.0	3.0	3.0	130
CAMPBELL'S CONDENSED						
Chicken (100g + water)	5	-	5	1.6	0.9	not known
Tomato (100g + water)	8.5	-	8.5	0.8	3.2	not known
CAMPBELLS, PREPARED FROM CONDENSED						
Beef Broth (250ml)	1.0	0.0	1.0	3.0	0.0	15
Cream of Celery (250ml)	10.0	1.0	9.0	2.0	5.0	90
Chicken broth (250ml)	2.0	0.0	2.0	2.0	2.0	30
Consomme, beef (250ml)	2.0	0.0	2.0	4.0	0.0	25
Cream of Chicken (250ml)	8.0	1.0	7.0	3.0	7.0	110
Golden Mushroom (250ml)	10.0	1.0	9.0	2.0	3.0	80
Green Pea (250ml)	29.0	5.0	24.0	9.0	3.0	180
Minestrone (250ml)	15.0	4.0	11.0	4.0	1.5	90
Tomato (250ml)	18.0	2.0	16.0	2.0	0.0	80
Vegetable (250ml)	16.0	2.0	14.0	3.0	1.0	90
Vegetable Beef (250ml)	13.0	2.0	11.0	4.0	1.5	80
Vegetarian Vegetable (250ml)	14.0	2.0	12.0	2.0	0.0	60
HEINZ						
Cream of tomato (200g)	14.2	0.8	13.4	1.7	7.2	not known
Cream of mushroom (200g)	10.2	0.2	10	2.8	5.5	not known
Cream of chicken + veg (200g)	12.4	1.3	11.1	2.3	1.9	not known

Food Item (Amount)	Carb (g)	Fibre (g)	Net Carbs (g)	Protein (g)	Fat (g)	Cals
Blended carrot + coriander (200g)	12.3	1.2	11.1	1.5	5.3	not known
French onion (200g)	10.9	0.9	10	0.9	0.1	not known
Country vegetable (200g)	18.6	2.2	16.4	4.6	0.9	not known
KNORR SOUP IN A CUP						
Beef Vegetable Soup (1)	27.0	1.0	26.0	5.0	2.0	150
Red Bean Chili (1)	32.0	8.0	24.0	9.0	1.0	170
LIPTON SOUP IN A CUP						
Beefy Mushroom (1)	6.6	0.1	6.5	0.9	0.4	33
Harvest Vegetable (1)	17.0	2.0	15.0	1.0	1.5	90
Vegetable (1)	6.5	1.0	5.5	0.8	0.2	28
SPINNAKER SEAFOOD						
Clam Chowder Soup (100g)	4.5	0.4	4.1	1.8	7	not known
Bouillabaisse (200g)	12.6	1.0	11.6	8.4	10.8	not known

FISH AND SHELLFISH

Most fish and shellfish have no carbohydrates, or very few. The notable exceptions are mussels, oysters and surimi (synthetic crabmeat). In addition to being low in carbs, salmon, sardines, mackerel and other fatty fish are good sources of omega-3 fatty acids.

Food Item (Amount)	Carb (g)	Fibre (g)	Net Carbs (g)	Protein (g)	Fat (g)	Cals
Fish						
BASS						
Sea Bass, baked (175g)	0.0	0.0	0.0	40.2	4.4	211
Striped Bass, baked (175g)	0.0	0.0	0.0	38.7	5.1	211
Bluefish, baked (175g)	0.0	0.0	0.0	43.7	9.3	270
Catfish, baked (175g)	0.0	0.0	0.0	31.8	13.6	259
COD						
Baked (175g)	0.0	0.0	0.0	38.8	1.5	179
Dried, salted (75g)	0.0	0.0	0.0	53.4	2.0	247
In batter (100g)	11.7	0.5	11.2	16.1	15.4	247
In breadcrumbs (100g)	15.2	0.4	14.8	12.4	14.3	235
Poached	Trace	0	Trace	20.9	1.1	94
Flounder, baked (175g)	0.0	0.0	0.0	41.1	2.6	199
HADDOCK						
Baked (175g)	0.0	0.0	0.0	40.7	1.6	187
In breadcrumbs (100g)	12.6	0.6	12.0	14.7	10.0	196

Food Item (Amount)	Carb (g)	Fibre (g)	Net Carbs (g)	Protein (g)	Fat (g)	Cals
Smoked (175g)	0.0	0.0	0.0	42.9	1.6	197
Steamed (100g)	0	0	0	20.9	0.6	89
Halibut, baked (175g)	0.0	0.0	0.0	45.4	5.0	238
Herring, grilled (100g)	0	0	0	20.1	11.2	181
Mackerel, baked (175g)	0.0	0.0	0.0	40.6	30.3	446
Mahi-mahi, baked (175g)	0.0	0.0	0.0	42.0	1.6	193
SALMON						
Baked (175g)	0.0	0.0	0.0	37.6	21.0	350
Tinned (175g)	0.0	0.0	0.0	34.8	12.4	260
Smoked (175g)	0.0	0.0	0.0	31.1	7.4	199
SARDINES						
Tinned in oil (175g)	0.0	0.0	0.0	41.9	19.5	354
Tinned in tomato sauce (175g)	0.0	0.0	0.0	27.8	20.4	303
Shad, baked (175g)	0.0	0.0	0.0	36.9	30.0	429
Snapper, baked (175g)	0.0	0.0	0.0	44.7	2.9	218
Swordfish, baked (175g)	0.0	0.0	0.0	43.2	8.7	264
Trout, baked (175g)	0.0	0.0	0.0	45.3	14.4	323
TUNA						
Baked (175g)	0.0	0.0	0.0	50.9	10.7	313
White, tinned in oil (175g)	0.0	0.0	0.0	45.1	13.7	316
White, tinned in water (175g)	0.0	0.0	0.0	40.2	5.1	218
Shellfish						
CLAMS						
Tinned, drained (175g)	8.7	0.0	8.7	43.5	3.3	252
Fried, (15 pieces)	20.0	0.0	20.0	8.0	15.0	250
CRAB						
Tinned, drained (175g)	0.0	0.0	0.0	34.9	2.1	168
Steamed (175g)	0.0	0.0	0.0	34.4	3.0	174

Food Item (Amount)	Carb (g)	Fibre (g)	Net Carbs (g)	Protein (g)	Fat (g)	Cals
Surimi (imitation crabmeat) (175g)	17.4	0.0	17.4	20.5	2.2	174
Crawfish (175g)	0.0	0.0	0.0	32.6	1.9	169
Lobster, steamed (175g)	2.2	0.0	2.2	34.9	1.0	167
Mussels, steamed (175g)	12.6	0.0	12.6	40.5	7.6	293
OYSTERS						
Tinned (175g)	6.7	0.0	6.7	12.0	4.2	117
Raw (175g)	6.7	0.0	6.7	12.0	4.2	116
Smoked (175g)	18.2	12.2	6.1	30.4	18.2	304
Prawns, steamed (175g)	0.0	0.0	0.0	35.6	1.8	168
SCALLOPS						
Baked (175g)	4.9	0.0	4.9	34.7	6.7	228
Fried (13 pieces)	27.0	1.0	26.0	12.0	7.0	220
SHRIMP						
Cocktail (175g)	15.7	3.6	12.0	20.8	1.9	161
Cooked (175g)	0.0	0.0	0.0	35.6	1.8	168
Squid, cooked (175g)	6.4	0.0	6.4	32.2	8.0	236

BEEF, PORK AND LAMB

The only high-carbohydrate items in this category are calf's liver and some luncheon meats, such as liverwurst and pastrami. Versatile and readily available, beef, pork and lamb are an important part of a controlled carbohydrate programme. This does not mean, however, that portions should be excessively large.

Food Item (Amount)	Carb (g)	Fibre (g)	Net Carbs (g)	Protein (g)	Fat (g)	Cals
Beef and Veal						
BEEF, ROASTED/COOKED						
Brisket (175g)	0.0	0.0	0.0	44.0	41.7	563
Chuck (175g)	0.0	0.0	0.0	50.1	31.6	498
Chuck eye steak (175g)	0.0	0.0	0.0	46.2	41.1	568
Corned beef brisket (175g)	0.3	0.0	0.3	33.3	33.8	449
Cubed steak (175g)	0.0	0.0	0.0	53.9	8.3	306
Eye round (175g)	0.0	0.0	0.0	45.3	24.0	410
Minced chuck (175g)	0.0	0.0	0.0	38.9	44.0	562
Minced round (175g)	0.0	0.0	0.0	46.7	28.1	454
Jerky (150g)	0.0	0.0	0.0	4.0	2.0	35
Prime rib (175g)	0.0	0.0	0.0	37.0	56.4	667
Rib eye roast (175g)	0.0	0.0	0.0	37.0	56.4	667
Rib eye steak (175g)	0.0	0.0	0.0	42.4	37.9	522
Roast (175g)	0.0	0.0	0.0	38.7	45.6	576
Roast, deli (175g)	2.3	0.0	2.3	34.4	5.2	193

Food Item (Amount)	Carb (g)	Fibre (g)	Net Carbs (g)	Protein (g)	Fat (g)	Cals
Shell steak (175g)	0.0	0.0	0.0	48.7	16.0	352
Short ribs (175g)	0.0	0.0	0.0	36.7	71.4	801
Sirloin steak (175g)	0.0	0.0	0.0	51.7	13.6	344
Skirt steak (175g)	0.0	0.0	0.0	46.2	41.1	568
Tenderloin (175g)	0.0	0.0	0.0	40.9	49.2	619
Top loin (175g)	0.0	0.0	0.0	51.7	12.3	332
Top sirloin (175g)	0.0	0.0	0.0	44.2	30.4	463
Liver, calf (175g)	10.4	0.0	10.4	40.5	9.9	304
VEAL, ROASTED/COOKED						
Breast (175g)	0.0	0.0	0.0	39.6	33.5	472
Cutlet (175g)	0.0	0.0	0.0	51.4	29.3	483
Escalopes (175g)	0.0	0.0	0.0	47.8	5.8	255
Loin (175g)	0.0	0.0	0.0	51.4	29.3	483
Minced (175g)	0.0	0.0	0.0	41.5	12.9	293
Rib chop (175g)	0.0	0.0	0.0	40.8	23.8	388
Round steak (175g)	0.0	0.0	0.0	47.6	7.0	265
Shank (175g)	0.0	0.0	0.0	43.4	7.9	256
Shoulder (175g)	0.0	0.0	0.0	43.3	14.0	311
Stew meat (175g)	0.0	0.0	0.0	40.2	13.4	292
Lamb and Goat						
Goat, roasted (175g)	0.0	0.0	0.0	46.1	5.2	243
LAMB, ROASTED						
Leg, bone-in (175g)	0.0	0.0	0.0	48.1	13.2	325
Minced (175g)	0.0	0.0	0.0	42.1	33.4	481
Rack, bone-in (175g)	0.0	0.0	0.0	44.5	22.6	395
Rib chop (175g)	0.0	0.0	0.0	37.6	50.3	614
Shoulder (175g)	0.0	0.0	0.0	48.1	13.2	325
Stew meat (175g)	0.0	0.0	0.0	57.3	15.0	379

Food Item (Amount)	Carb (g)	Fibre (g)	Net Carbs (g)	Protein (g)	Fat (g)	Cals
Lunch Meats and Sausage						
Bologna, beef (3 slices)	2.0	0.0	2.0	9.3	24.5	266
Bologna, beef & pork (3 slices)	2.4	0.0	2.4	10.0	24.1	269
Breakfast sausage (1)	1.2	0.7	0.5	4.5	1.0	32
Chorizo (50g)	1.1	0.0	1.1	13.7	21.7	258
FRANKFURTER						
Beef & pork (50g)	1.5	0.0	1.5	6.8	17.0	188
Beef (1)	1.2	0.0	1.2	5.0	13.1	143
Ham (175g)	1.8	0.0	1.8	28.2	6.6	174
Liverwurst (175g)	9.6	3.0	6.6	21.6	43.2	528
Pastrami, beef (175g)	5.2	0.0	5.2	29.3	49.6	594
Pepperoni (5 pieces)	0.8	0.0	0.8	5.8	12.1	137
Pork and beef sausage (1)	0.7	0.0	0.7	3.7	9.8	107
Pork sausage (1)	1.0	0.0	1.0	13.4	17.2	216
Spam (50g)	0.8	0.0	0.8	7.4	15.8	174
SALAMI						
Beef (3 pieces)	1.9	0.0	1.9	10.4	14.3	181
Beef and pork (3 pieces)	0.8	0.0	0.8	6.9	10.3	125
Pork (3 pieces)	0.5	0.0	0.5	6.8	10.1	122
Pork						
PORK, ROASTED/COOKED						
Bacon (3 pieces)	0.1	0.0	0.1	5.8	9.4	109
Chop, centre cut, bone-in (175g)	0.0	0.0	0.0	50.7	14.1	344
Frankfurter (1)	1.5	0.0	1.5	6.4	16.5	181
Minced (175g)	0.0	0.0	0.0	43.7	35.3	505
Ham, boneless (175g)	0.0	0.0	0.0	38.5	15.3	303
Loin chop, bone-in (175g)	0.0	0.0	0.0	37.3	43.3	549

Food Item (Amount)	Carb (g)	Fibre (g)	Net Carbs (g)	Protein (g)	Fat (g)	Cals
Loin roast (175g)	0.0	0.0	0.0	46.1	24.9	422
Pancetta (25g)	0.2	0.0	0.2	8.6	14.0	163
Prosciutto (175g)	0.9	0.0	0.9	37.4	13.0	281
Sausage, Italian (50g)	0.9	0.0	0.9	11.4	14.6	183
Spareribs (175g)	0.0	0.0	0.0	49.4	51.5	675
Tenderloin (175g)	0.0	0.0	0.0	47.9	8.2	279

POULTRY

Barbecued, baked or grilled poultry is virtually carb free. Just be careful with seasonings and cooking methods: adding breadcrumbs, batter, sweet and sour sauces, glazes, barbecue sauces, pastry crusts and sweet dips all sneak in carbs. In general, whether dining out or eating in, the simpler the better.

Food Item (Amount)	Carb (g)	Fibre (g)	Net Carbs (g)	Protein (g)	Fat (g)	Cals
Chicken						
Chicken breast in breadcrumbs (fried) (100g)	14.8	0.7	14.1	18.0	12.7	242
Chicken burger (inc. bun, mayonnaise) (100g)	23.4	Trace	23.4	12.5	10.8	267
Chicken chasseur (100g)	2.3	0.3	2.0	12.8	4.1	97
Chicken chow mein (100g)	12.7	1.1	11.6	8.5	7.2	147
Chicken curry (takeaway) (100g)	2.5	0.8	1.7	11.7	9.8	145
Chicken in white sauce (tinned) (100g)	2.5	Trace	2.5	14.3	8.3	141
Chicken pie (100g)	24.6	0.8	23.8	9.0	17.7	288
Chicken roll (100g)	5.2	Trace	5.2	17.1	4.8	131
Chicken satay (100g)	3.0	2.2	0.8	21.7	10.3	191
Chicken stir-fried with rice + vegetables (100g)	17.1	1.3	15.8	6.5	4.6	132
Chicken tandoori (100g)	2.0	Trace	2.0	27.4	10.8	214

Food Item (Amount)	Carb (g)	Fibre (g)	Net Carbs (g)	Protein (g)	Fat (g)	Cals
Chicken tikka masala (100g)	2.6	1.6	1.0	12.9	10.6	157
Chicken wings, marinated, barbecued (100g)	4.1	Trace	4.1	27.4	16.6	274
Coq au vin (100g)	3.2	0.3	2.9	11.1	11.0	155
CHICKEN, ROASTED						
Breast fillet, skinless (175g)	0.0	0.0	0.0	50.7	13.2	335
Breast, with skin, boneless (175g)	0.0	0.0	0.0	50.7	13.2	335
Drumstick, skinless, boneless (175g)	0.0	0.0	0.0	48.1	9.6	293
Drumstick, with skin (175g)	0.0	0.0	0.0	46.0	19.0	367
Minced (175g)	0.0	0.0	0.0	49.2	12.6	323
Leg, boneless, with skin (175g)	0.0	0.0	0.0	44.2	22.9	395
Light and dark (175g)	0.0	0.0	0.0	40.8	22.8	379
Thigh, boneless, with skin (175g)	0.0	0.0	0.0	42.6	26.4	420
Wing, boneless (175g)	0.0	0.0	0.0	45.7	33.1	493
CHICKEN, REFRIGERATED, PREPARED						
Roasted Whole Chicken (75g)	1.0	0.0	1.0	16.0	11.0	160
Cornish hen, roasted (175g)	0.0	0.0	0.0	37.9	31.0	442
Duck and Goose						
DUCK, ROASTED						
Breast, without skin (175g)	0.0	0.0	0.0	45.0	9.6	279
Crispy duck, Chinese style (takeaway) (100g)	0.3	0	0.3	27.9	24.2	331
Whole (175g)	0.0	0.0	0.0	26.1	89.2	916
Goose, roasted (175g)	0.0	0.0	0.0	42.8	37.3	519
Pheasant (roast) (100g)	0	0	0	27.9	12.0	220

Food Item (Amount)	Carb (g)	Fibre (g)	Net Carbs (g)	Protein (g)	Fat (g)	Cals
Turkey						
TURKEY, ROASTED						
Breast, without skin (175g)	0.0	0.0	0.0	51.1	1.3	230
Minced (175g)	0.0	0.0	0.0	46.5	22.4	400
Light and dark (175g)	0.1	0.0	0.1	47.6	16.1	349
Sausage (50g)	0.3	0.0	0.3	9.6	6.4	97

NUTS, NUT BUTTERS AND SEEDS

Nuts and seeds are high in protein, fibre, flavour and fat – which makes a small handful a filling, nutritional and energizing snack. Macadamias, walnuts, pecans and Brazil nuts are top choices because they have a higher fat content and are lower in carbs than other nuts. Add a small amount of chopped nuts for a nice crunch in casseroles and extra flavour in vegetable side dishes. They're also an important ingredient in controlled carb desserts: finely ground nuts often take the place of white flour.

Food Item (Amount)	Carb (g)	Fibre (g)	Net Carbs (g)	Protein (g)	Fat (g)	Cals
ALMONDS						
Butter (2tbs)	6.8	1.2	5.6	4.8	18.9	203
Paste (25g)	13.6	1.4	12.2	2.6	7.9	130
Slivered, blanched (2tbs)	3.3	1.6	1.7	3.5	8.6	102
Whole, roasted (24)	5.7	3.4	2.3	6.1	14.6	166
Brazil nuts, roasted (6)	3.6	1.5	2.1	4.1	18.8	186
CASHEWS						
Butter (2tbs)	8.8	0.6	8.2	5.6	15.8	188
Whole, roasted (2tbs)	5.6	0.5	5.1	2.6	7.9	98
Chestnuts, roasted (6)	26.7	2.6	24.2	1.6	1.1	124
Coconut, dried, unsweetened (2tbs)	2.4	1.6	0.8	0.7	6.3	64
Hazelnuts, roasted (2tbs)	2.8	1.6	1.2	2.5	10.3	106

Food Item (Amount)	Carb (g)	Fibre (g)	Net Carbs (g)	Protein (g)	Fat (g)	Cals
MACADAMIA NUTS						
Butter (2tbs)	5.0	0.0	5.0	3.0	24.0	230
Roasted (2tbs)	2.3	1.4	0.9	1.3	12.7	120
Nutella (2tbs)	23.0	2.0	21.0	3.0	10.0	200
PEANUTS						
Butter, crunchy (2tbs)	6.9	2.1	4.8	7.7	15.9	187
Butter, smooth (2tbs)	6.2	1.9	4.3	8.1	16.3	190
Oil-roasted (2tbs)	3.4	1.7	1.8	4.7	8.9	105
Pecans, roasted (2tbs)	1.9	1.3	0.6	1.2	9.7	93
Pine nuts (2tbs)	2.4	0.8	1.7	4.1	8.6	96
Pistachios (2tbs)	4.7	1.6	3.1	3.3	6.9	88
Pumpkin seeds, hulled (2tbs)	4.3	0.3	4.0	1.5	1.6	36
Sesame seeds (2tbs)	4.2	2.1	2.1	3.2	8.9	103
Soya beans, roasted (2tbs)	7.0	1.7	5.3	8.5	4.7	97
Sunflower seeds, hulled (2tbs)	3.9	1.8	2.1	3.1	8.0	93
Walnuts, halves (2tbs)	1.7	0.8	0.9	1.9	8.2	82

VEGETABLES

Potatoes are one of the most popular vegetables in the UK, but they should be at the bottom of your option list. In terms of nutritional density, dark green vegetables rate number one in antioxidant capacity, and cruciferous vegetables, such as cabbage, broccoli or Brussels sprouts, are known to help fight disease. Cooked kale or spinach topped with toasted garlic and olive oil is delicious, as well as among the most healthful foods you can eat. On Lifetime Maintenance, most people can also enjoy moderate portions of higher glycemic veggies such as winter squash, carrots and sweet potatoes, all of which are loaded with beta-carotene.

Food Item (Amount)	Carb (g)	Fibre (g)	Net Carbs (g)	Protein (g)	Fat (g)	Cals
ARTICHOKES						
Whole (1)	13.4	6.5	6.9	4.2	0.2	60
Hearts, frozen (2tbs)	7.8	6.0	1.8	2.7	0.4	38
Hearts, marinated (4 pieces)	4.0	2.0	2.0	0.0	4.0	40
ASPARAGUS						
Steamed (4 spears)	2.5	1.0	1.6	1.6	0.2	14
Tinned (4 pieces)	1.8	1.2	0.6	1.5	0.5	14
Frozen, steamed (2tbs)	4.4	1.4	2.9	2.7	0.4	25
Aubergine, grilled (2tbs)	3.3	1.2	2.1	0.4	0.1	14

Food Item (Amount)	Carb (g)	Fibre (g)	Net Carbs (g)	Protein (g)	Fat (g)	Cals
Bamboo shoots, tinned, sliced (2tbs)	2.1	0.9	1.2	1.1	0.3	12
BEANS						
Broad, steamed (2tbs)	16.7	4.6	12.1	6.5	0.3	94
Green, steamed (2tbs)	4.9	2.0	2.9	1.2	0.2	22
Yellow wax, steamed (2tbs)	4.9	2.1	2.9	1.2	0.2	22
Beets, tinned (2tbs)	6.1	1.4	4.7	0.8	0.1	26
Bok choi (2tbs)	1.5	1.4	0.2	1.3	0.1	10
BROCCOLI						
Florets, raw (2tbs)	1.9	1.1	0.8	1.1	0.1	10
Frozen, chopped, steamed (2tbs)	4.9	2.8	2.2	2.9	0.1	26
Brussels sprouts, steamed (2tbs)	6.8	2.0	4.7	2.0	0.4	30
CABBAGE						
Chinese (2tbs)	1.4	1.4	0.0	0.9	0.1	8
Green, shredded, raw (2tbs)	1.9	0.8	1.1	0.5	0.1	9
Green, steamed (2tbs)	3.3	1.7	1.6	0.8	0.3	17
Red, shredded, raw (2tbs)	2.1	0.7	1.4	0.5	0.1	9
Savoy, steamed (2tbs)	3.9	2.0	1.9	1.3	0.1	17
Cardoon, steamed (2tbs)	3.9	1.2	2.7	0.6	0.1	16
CARROT						
Sliced, steamed (2tbs)	8.2	2.6	5.6	0.9	0.1	35
Whole, 19cm long, raw (1)	7.3	2.2	5.1	0.7	0.1	31
Cassava, cooked (2tbs)	26.3	1.3	25.1	0.9	0.2	111
CAULIFLOWER						
Raw (2tbs)	2.6	1.3	1.4	1.0	0.1	13
Steamed (2tbs)	2.6	1.7	0.9	1.1	0.3	14

Food Item (Amount)	Carb (g)	Fibre (g)	Net Carbs (g)	Protein (g)	Fat (g)	Cals
Cauliflower cheese (skimmed milk) (100g)	5.1	1.3	3.8	6.0	6.5	102
CELERY						
Steamed (2tbs)	3.0	1.2	1.8	0.6	0.1	14
Raw (1 stick)	1.5	0.7	0.8	0.3	0.1	6
Celeriac, cooked (2tbs)	4.6	0.9	3.6	0.7	0.2	21
Chard, steamed (2tbs)	3.6	1.8	1.8	1.7	0.1	18
Chicory (2tbs)	1.8	1.4	0.4	0.4	0.1	8
Coleslaw, with dressing (2tbs)	7.5	0.9	6.6	0.8	1.6	41
CORN						
Tinned (2tbs)	15.2	1.6	13.6	2.2	0.8	66
Cob (1)	19.3	2.2	17.2	2.6	1.0	83
Cream style, tinned (2tbs)	23.2	1.5	21.7	2.2	0.5	92
Kernels (2tbs)	14.7	2.1	12.6	2.5	0.9	66
Cucumber slices (2tbs)	1.4	0.4	1.0	0.4	0.1	7
Dandelion greens (2tbs)	3.4	1.5	1.8	1.1	0.3	17
FENNEL						
Braised (2tbs)	2.8	1.3	1.5	0.6	0.1	12
Raw (2tbs)	3.2	1.4	1.8	0.5	0.1	13
Garlic cloves (1)	1.0	0.1	0.9	0.2	0.0	4
Jerusalem artichoke, raw (2tbs)	13.1	1.2	11.9	1.5	0.0	57
Kale, steamed (2tbs)	3.4	1.3	2.1	1.9	0.3	20
Kohlrabi, steamed (2tbs)	5.5	0.9	4.6	1.5	0.1	24
LETTUCE						
Iceberg (small handful)	0.6	0.4	0.2	0.3	0.1	3
Romaine (small handful)	0.7	0.5	0.2	0.5	0.1	4
Marrow (100g)	1.6	0.6	1.0	0.4	0.2	9

Food Item (Amount)	Carb (g)	Fibre (g)	Net Carbs (g)	Protein (g)	Fat (g)	Cals
MUSHROOMS						
Garlic mushrooms (not coated) (100g)	0.7	1.2	0.5	2.1	14.4	140
Portabella (100g)	5.8	1.7	4.1	2.8	0.2	29
Shiitake, cooked (2tbs)	10.4	1.5	8.8	1.1	0.2	40
Straw, tinned (2tbs)	4.2	2.3	2.0	3.5	0.6	29
Whole, raw (2tbs)	2.0	0.6	1.4	1.4	0.2	12
Mustard greens, steamed (2tbs)	1.5	1.4	0.1	1.6	0.2	11
Okra, steamed (2tbs)	5.8	2.0	3.8	1.5	0.1	26
Onions, chopped, raw (2tbs)	6.9	1.4	5.5	0.9	0.1	30
Parsley, chopped (1tbs)	0.2	0.1	0.1	0.1	0.0	1
Parsnips, steamed (2tbs)	15.2	3.1	12.1	1.0	0.2	63
PEAS						
Frozen (2tbs)	9.9	3.4	6.5	3.8	0.3	55
Mange tout (100g)	3.3	2.3	1.0	3.2	0.1	26
Mushy (100g)	13.8	1.8	12.0	5.8	0.7	81
Pea pods (2tbs)	5.6	2.2	3.4	2.6	0.2	34
PEPPERS						
Green, raw (2tbs)	4.8	1.3	3.5	0.7	0.1	20
Red, raw (2tbs)	4.8	1.5	3.3	0.7	0.1	20
POTATO						
Baked, small (½)	11.6	1.1	10.5	1.1	0.1	50
Boiled (2tbs)	15.6	1.4	14.2	1.3	0.1	67
Croquettes (100g)	21.6	1.3	20.3	3.7	13.1	214
French fries, frozen (10)	15.8	2.0	13.9	1.6	3.8	101
Fritters (100g)	25.5	1.5	24	3.2	8.5	185
Hash browns, frozen, cooked (2tbs)	21.9	1.6	20.4	2.5	9.0	170

Food Item (Amount)	Carb (g)	Fibre (g)	Net Carbs (g)	Protein (g)	Fat (g)	Cals
Mashed, from flakes, prepared (2tbs)	15.8	2.4	13.4	2.0	5.9	119
Salad (with mayonnaise) (100g)	11.4	0.8	10.6	1.5	26.5	287
Waffles	30.3	2.3	28	3.2	8.2	200
PUMPKIN						
Boiled (2)	6.0	1.4	4.6	0.9	0.1	25
Tinned (2tbs)	9.2	5.1	4.1	2.1	0.0	41
Radicchio (2tbs)	0.9	0.2	0.7	0.3	0.1	5
Radishes (10)	1.6	0.7	0.9	0.3	0.2	9
Ratatouille (100g)	3.7	1.0	2.7	1.2	6.6	78
Rutabaga, boiled (2tbs)	7.4	1.5	5.9	1.1	0.2	33
Sauerkraut (2tbs)	5.1	3.0	2.1	1.1	0.2	22
Shallots (2tbs)	13.4	0.6	12.9	2.0	0.1	58
Sorrel, cooked (2tbs)	1.5	1.3	0.2	0.9	0.3	10
SPINACH						
Frozen, steamed (2tbs)	5.1	2.9	2.2	3.0	0.2	27
Raw (2tbs)	0.5	0.4	0.1	0.4	0.1	3
Spring onions (2tbs)	3.7	1.3	2.4	0.9	0.1	16
SPROUTS, RAW						
Alfalfa (2tbs)	0.6	0.4	0.2	0.7	0.1	5
Bean (2tbs)	3.1	1.0	2.1	1.6	0.0	16
SQUASH						
Acorn, baked (2tbs)	14.9	4.5	10.4	1.2	0.1	57
Acorn, boiled (2tbs)	10.8	3.2	7.6	0.8	0.1	42
Butternut, baked, cubes (2tbs)	10.8	2.9	7.9	0.9	0.1	41
Butternut, baked, mashed (2tbs)	12.9	3.4	9.4	1.1	0.1	49

Food Item (Amount)	Carb (g)	Fibre (g)	Net Carbs (g)	Protein (g)	Fat (g)	Cals
Courgettes, raw (2tbs)	1.9	0.8	1.1	0.8	0.1	9
Courgettes, steamed (2tbs)	2.6	1.1	1.5	1.1	0.1	13
Spaghetti, cooked (2tbs)	5.0	1.1	3.9	0.5	0.2	21
Summer/Yellow, raw (2tbs)	2.5	1.1	1.4	0.7	0.1	11
Summer/Yellow, steamed (2tbs)	3.9	1.3	2.6	0.8	0.3	18
SWEET POTATO						
Baked, medium (½)	13.8	1.7	12.1	1.0	0.1	59
Boiled (½)	18.3	1.4	17.0	1.3	0.2	79
Mashed (2tbs)	39.8	3.0	36.9	2.7	0.5	172
TOMATO						
Cherry (10)	7.9	1.9	6.0	1.4	0.6	36
Plum (1)	2.9	0.7	2.2	0.5	0.2	13
Small (75g)	4.2	1.0	3.2	0.8	0.3	19
Sun-dried, in oil (2tbs)	3.2	0.8	2.4	0.7	1.9	29
TOMATO PRODUCTS, TINNED						
Diced, in juice (1tbs)	2.5	0.5	2.0	0.5	0.0	13
Paste (2tbs)	6.3	1.3	5.0	1.2	0.2	27
Puree (2tbs)	3.0	0.6	2.4	0.5	0.1	13
TURNIP GREENS						
Frozen, chopped (2tbs)	3.0	2.1	1.0	2.0	0.3	18
Fresh, steamed (2tbs)	3.1	2.5	0.6	0.8	0.2	14
TURNIPS						
Boiled, cubes (2tbs)	3.8	1.6	2.3	0.6	0.1	16
Boiled, mashed (2tbs)	5.6	2.3	3.3	0.8	0.1	24
Vegeburger (100g)	8.0	4.2	3.8	16.6	11.1	196
Vegetable and cheese burger in crumbs (100g)	23.0	1.6	21.4	7.0	14.0	240

Food Item (Amount)	Carb (g)	Fibre (g)	Net Carbs (g)	Protein (g)	Fat (g)	Cals
Vegetable and rice salad (100g)	23.1	0.7	22.4	3.0	7.5	165
Vegetables and tagliatelle (100g)	11.0	0.7	10.3	1.6	3.0	74
Vegetable bake (100g)	13.1	1.2	11.9	4.3	7.2	131
Vegetable Kiev (100g)	17.6	1.2	16.4	9.9	13.7	229
Vegetable pasty (100g)	33.1	2.0	31.1	4.0	16.5	289
Vegetable pie (100g)	18.8	1.5	17.3	3.0	8.4	159
Vegetable samosa (100g)	30.0	2.5	27.5	5.1	9.3	217
Vegetable shepherd's pie (100g)	13.3	1.2	12.1	1.9	14.9	101
Waterchestnuts (2tbs)	8.7	1.8	7.0	0.6	0.0	35
Watercress (2tbs)	0.2	0.2	0.0	0.4	0.0	2
Yams, tinned, mashed (2tbs)	29.7	2.2	27.5	2.5	0.3	129

GRAINS, PASTA AND RICE

Bland, chewy and comforting, grains, pasta and rice are permitted in moderation once you're close to your goal weight. Whole grain varieties, which are high in fibre, are preferable nutritionally to processed grains (i.e. brown rice instead of white rice). Some grains, such as buckwheat, bulgar and wheatgerm, are high in protein. Look for controlled carb pastas and other grain dishes.

Food Item (Amount)	Carb (g)	Fibre (g)	Net Carbs (g)	Protein (g)	Fat (g)	Cals
Grains						
Barley, cooked (2tbs)	22.2	3.0	19.2	1.8	0.4	97
BRAN						
Oat (2tbs)	7.8	1.8	6.0	2.0	0.8	29
Wheat (2tbs)	4.7	3.1	1.6	1.1	0.3	16
Bulgar, cooked (2tbs)	16.9	4.1	12.8	2.8	0.2	76
Cornmeal (2tbs)	13.4	1.3	12.1	1.5	0.3	63
Kasha (buckwheat groats), cooked (2tbs)	74.3	9.4	64.8	11.6	2.7	343
Masa (corn flour) (2tbs)	10.9	1.4	9.5	1.3	0.5	52
Millet, cooked (2tbs)	28.4	1.6	26.8	4.2	1.2	143
Quinoa, dry (1tbs)	29.3	2.5	26.8	5.6	2.5	159
Tabbouleh, dry (1tbs)	26.0	6.0	20.0	4.0	0.5	120
Pasta and Couscous						
Couscous, cooked (4oz)	18.2	1.1	17.1	3.0	0.1	88

Food Item (Amount)	Carb (g)	Fibre (g)	Net Carbs (g)	Protein (g)	Fat (g)	Cals
NOODLES, COOKED						
Egg (2tbs)	19.9	0.9	19.0	3.8	1.2	106
Japanese somen (2tbs)	24.2	1.4	22.8	3.5	0.2	115
Rice (2tbs)	21.9	0.9	21.0	0.8	0.2	96
Thai rice (2tbs)	24.5	1.0	23.5	1.5	0.1	105
Udon (brown rice), dry (25g)	19.6	1.6	18.0	4.1	1.0	103
PASTA, COOKED						
Fresh (100g)	28.3	2.0	26.3	5.8	1.2	149
Macaroni (2tbs)	17.8	0.9	16.9	5.1	0.1	94
Plain, all shapes (2tbs)	19.8	0.9	18.9	3.3	0.5	99
Ravioli, frozen (4)	40.0	2.0	38.0	12.0	6.0	260
Spinach (2tbs)	18.3	2.5	15.9	3.2	0.4	91
Wholewheat (2tbs)	18.6	2.0	16.6	3.7	0.4	87
PASTA, SPECIALITY, COOKED						
Corn (2tbs)	22.5	3.1	19.4	2.1	0.6	101
Quinoa (2tbs)	17.5	1.2	16.3	2.0	1.0	90
Rice (2tbs)	23.5	1.5	22.0	1.0	0.0	92
Semolina (2tbs)	20.6	1.0	19.7	3.8	0.7	102
Sesame rice (2tbs)	18.5	2.0	16.5	4.0	1.0	100
Spelt (2tbs)	20.0	2.5	17.5	4.0	0.8	95
PASTA DISHES						
Lasagne	14.6	0.8	13.8	9.8	10.8	191
Macaroni cheese	12.2	0.5	11.7	6.7	9.9	162
Ravioli, beef in tomato and meat sauce, tinned (4tbs)	36.9	3.7	33.2	8.4	5.4	229
Spaghetti bolognese	5.3	0.9	4.4	9.3	5.7	108
Vegetables and tagliatelle	11.0	0.7	10.3	1.6	3.0	74

Food Item (Amount)	Carb (g)	Fibre (g)	Net Carbs (g)	Protein (g)	Fat (g)	Cals
Spaghetti, w/tomato sauce & cheese, tinned (2tbs)	19.3	1.3	18.0	2.8	0.8	95

Rice

RICE, COOKED

Food Item (Amount)	Carb (g)	Fibre (g)	Net Carbs (g)	Protein (g)	Fat (g)	Cals
Basmati, dry (2tbs)	39.2	1.1	38.0	4.0	0.7	179
Brown (4tbs)	22.4	1.8	20.6	2.5	0.9	108
Egg fried rice (takeaway) (100g)	33.3	0.8	32.5	4.3	4.9	186
Pilau, plain (100g)	24.8	0.3	24.5	2.3	4.6	142
Short-grain risotto (4tbs)	26.7	0.9	25.8	2.2	0.2	121
White (4tbs)	22.3	0.3	21.9	2.1	0.2	103
Wild (4tbs)	17.5	1.5	16.0	3.3	0.3	83

PULSES, LEGUMES AND TOFU

Tofu is permitted in Induction, but you should not add beans and legumes back into your diet until you are well into OWL or even in the Pre-Maintenance phase. High in fibre, protein and a variety of minerals and vitamins, beans and other legumes are composed of carbohydrates with a fairly low glycemic index (although they vary from type to type). This means that they are digested relatively slowly, making you feel fuller longer. And unlike carbs with a higher glycemic index, which raise your blood-sugar level quickly, beans and other legumes are slowly absorbed in the bloodstream. Tofu and other soya products are known to help lower cholesterol and, in moderation, can be helpful for women in menopause. On a culinary note, beans, legumes and especially tofu are bland, so spice them up!

Food Item (Amount)	Carb (g)	Fibre (g)	Net Carbs (g)	Protein (g)	Fat (g)	Cals
Pulses and Legumes						
BAKED BEANS						
Plain (100g)	15.3	3.7	11.6	5.2	0.6	84
with pork (2tbs)	25.3	7.0	18.3	6.6	2.0	134
Vegetarian (2tbs)	26.1	6.4	19.7	6.1	0.6	118
Beans w/pork & tomato sauce, tinned (2tbs)	24.5	6.1	18.5	6.5	1.3	124
Black Beans (2tbs)	20.4	7.5	12.9	7.6	0.5	114

Food Item (Amount)	Carb (g)	Fibre (g)	Net Carbs (g)	Protein (g)	Fat (g)	Cals
Black-eyed peas (½ cup)	17.9	5.6	12.3	6.7	0.5	100
Chickpeas (2tbs)	20.0	7.0	13.0	5.0	2.5	120
CHILI, TINNED						
Con carne w/beans (2tbs)	14.1	4.7	9.4	11.6	4.7	147
Vegetarian w/beans (2tbs)	19.0	4.9	14.1	6.0	0.4	103
Falafel (50g patty)	18.1	3.2	14.9	7.6	10.1	189
Hummus (2tbs)	6.2	1.6	4.6	1.5	2.6	53
Kidney beans (2tbs)	19.8	8.2	11.6	8.1	0.1	110
Lentils (2tbs)	19.9	7.8	12.1	8.9	0.4	115
Lima beans, baby (2tbs)	21.2	7.0	14.2	7.3	0.4	115
Navy beans (2tbs)	23.9	5.8	18.1	7.9	0.5	129
Peas, split (2tbs)	20.7	8.1	12.6	8.2	0.4	116
Pink beans (2tbs)	23.6	4.5	19.1	7.7	0.4	126
Pinto beans (2tbs)	21.9	7.4	14.6	7.0	0.4	117
Refried beans, tinned (2tbs)	19.6	6.7	12.9	6.9	1.6	118
Soya beans, green (2tbs)	10.0	3.8	6.2	11.1	5.8	127
Tofu						
Firm (2tbs)	5.4	2.9	2.5	19.9	11.0	183
Regular (2tbs)	2.3	0.4	2.0	10.0	5.9	94

DESSERTS

Products especially made for individuals following a controlled carb programme are your best bet here. In second place are sugar-free desserts (though many contain milk, which is high in carbs). Even when desserts are low in carbohydrates, it's important to keep in mind that you need not eat one at the end of every meal. Set a weekly limit for yourself and stick to it. In nutritional terms, a handful of fresh berries with a dollop of whipped cream is always your best choice.

Food Item (Amount)	Carb (g)	Fibre (g)	Net Carbs (g)	Protein (g)	Fat (g)	Cals
Pudding						
Banana, made with whole milk (2tbs)	28.8	0.0	28.8	4.0	4.3	166
Chocolate, made with whole milk (2tbs)	27.6	1.5	26.2	4.6	4.6	163
Egg custard, made with whole milk (2tbs)	23.4	0.0	23.4	5.5	5.5	162
Rice, made with 2% milk (2tbs)	30.0	0.0	30.0	5.0	2.5	160
Tapioca, made with whole milk (2tbs)	27.6	0.0	27.6	4.1	4.1	161
Vanilla, made with whole milk (2tbs)	28.0	0.0	28.0	3.8	4.1	162

Food Item (Amount)	Carb (g)	Fibre (g)	Net Carbs (g)	Protein (g)	Fat (g)	Cals
READY-MADE PUDDING						
Banoffee pie (100g)	32.9	2.5	30.4	3.8	20.0	319
Cheesecake (100 g)	35.2	0.8	34.4	4.0	16.2	294
Creme Caramel (100g)	21.1	0.0	21.1	0.9	2.5	102
Creme Fraiche (30ml serving)	2.8	0.0	2.8	4.0	2.3	380
Custard, fresh 30g	3.8	0.0	3.8	4.9	0.8	621
Fruit trifle (100g)	19.5	2.1	17.4	2.6	9.0	164
Pavlova (100g)	42.2	0.3	41.9	2.7	13.2	288
Torte (100g)	27.7	0.5	27.2	3.8	15.5	258
Yeo Valley organic Pot au Chocolat (100g)	13.9	0.0	13.9	33.7	3.9	374
Sorbet						
HÄAGEN-DAZS						
Chocolate (2tbs)	28.0	2.0	26.0	2.0	0.0	120
Raspberry (2tbs)	30.0	2.0	28.0	0.0	0.0	120
Zesty Lemon (2tbs)	31.0	0.5	30.5	0.0	0.0	120
Whipped Topping						
Tip Top dessert topping (100g)	9.0	Trace	9.0	4.9	6.5	112
Dream Topping (100g)	12.2	Trace	9.0	3.9	11.7	166
Frozen Yogurt						
BEN & JERRY'S						
Cherry Garcia (2tbs)	31.0	0.0	31.0	4.0	3.0	170
Chocolate Fudge Brownie (2tbs)	36.0	1.0	35.0	6.0	3.0	190
HÄAGEN-DAZS						
Chocolate (2tbs)	28.0	0.8	27.3	6.0	0.0	140
Vanilla (2tbs)	29.0	0.0	29.0	6.0	0.0	140

Food Item (Amount)	Carb (g)	Fibre (g)	Net Carbs (g)	Protein (g)	Fat (g)	Cals
Ice Cream						
BEN & JERRY'S						
Cherry Garcia (2tbs)	25.0	0.0	25.0	4.0	16.0	240
Chocolate Chip Cookie Dough (2tbs)	30.0	0.0	30.0	4.0	17.0	270
Chocolate Fudge Brownie (2tbs)	33.0	2.0	31.0	4.0	14.0	250
NY Fudge Crunch (2tbs)	28.0	2.0	26.0	5.0	20.0	290
Cornetto	28.8	0.3	28.5	4.0	17.8	284
Chocolate nut sundae	26.2	0.2	26	2.6	14.9	243
HAAGEN-DAZS						
Chocolate (2tbs)	22.0	1.0	21.0	5.0	18.0	270
Coffee (2tbs)	21.0	0.0	21.0	5.0	18.0	270
Rum Raisin (2tbs)	22.0	0.0	22.0	4.0	17.0	270
Strawberry (2tbs)	23.0	0.8	22.3	4.0	16.0	250
Lollies, with ice cream	20.9	0	20.9	1.4	3.8	118
Lollies, with fruit juice	18.6	0	18.6	0.1	0.3	73
Mars, Bounty, Snickers ice cream bars	21.8	Trace	21.8	5.0	23.3	311
Vanilla, non-dairy	18.8	Trace	18.8	3.0	7.8	153
Viennetta	21.0	Trace	21.0	3.5	17.6	251
Mousse						
Cadbury's light 55g pot chocolate mousse	9.5	0.0	9.5	1.8	3.4	70
From instant (2tbs)	23.0	0.0	23.0	5.0	9.0	190

Food Item (Amount)	Carb (g)	Fibre (g)	Net Carbs (g)	Protein (g)	Fat (g)	Cals
Non-Dairy						
Rice Dream Vanilla Non-Dairy Dessert (2tbs)	23.0	1.0	22.0	0.0	6.0	150
Sorbet, various flavours (2tbs)	30.1	0.0	30.1	1.1	2.0	137
Miscellaneous Frozen Treats						
Frozen fruit bar, most flavours (75g)	18.6	0.0	18.6	1.1	0.0	75
Frozen fruit bar with cream (50g)	19.3	0.1	19.2	1.0	1.3	86

CAKES AND PIES

Occasionally, on Lifetime Maintenance, you might splurge on a small slice of pie or piece of cake. When you do so, make sure that you choose the best quality, so that a small portion satisfies you. And do note that some cakes and pies are lower in carbs than others: they contain less flour, less sugar and more fibre.

Food Item (Amount)	Carb (g)	Fibre (g)	Net Carbs (g)	Protein (g)	Fat (g)	Cals
Cake						
Banana bread (100g)	52.7	1.5	51.2	4.4	13.6	338
Battenburg cake (100g)	53.1	0.9	52.2	5.6	16.8	373
Black forest gateau (100g)	37.2	1.0	52.2	5.6	15.7	295
Carrot cake with topping (100g)	37.0	1.0	36	4.3	22.7	359
Cheesecake ($^1/_{12}$ cake)	20.4	0.3	20.1	4.4	18.0	257
Chocolate fudge cake (100g)	55.7	0.9	54.8	5.2	14.3	358
Chocolate pudding, from mix ($^1/_{12}$ cake)	34.2	1.5	32.7	3.5	14.3	270
Crispie cakes (100g)	73.8	1.9	71.9	5.7	18.0	461
Entenmann's Chocolate Fudge Cake (1 slice)	47.0	2.0	45.0	3.0	14.0	310
Entenmann's Sour Cream Chip & Nut Loaf (1 slice)	28.0	0.5	27.5	3.0	14.0	240

Food Item (Amount)	Carb (g)	Fibre (g)	Net Carbs (g)	Protein (g)	Fat (g)	Cals
Fruit & cream sponge gateau (100g)	33.3	0.9	32.4	3.2	12.3	248
Gingerbread, from mix (¹/₉ cake)	34.0	0.8	33.2	2.7	6.8	207
Jaffa Cakes (100g)	76.9	1.3	75.6	4.0	8.1	377
Madeira cake w/butter (¹/₁₂ cake)	13.8	0.1	13.7	1.6	5.6	110
Madeira cake (100g)	58.4	0.9	57.5	5.4	15.1	377
Muffins, America-style, chocolate chip (100g)	52.3	1.6	50.7	6.3	18.2	385
Rich fruit cake (100g)	59.9	1.5	58.4	3.9	11.4	343
Rich fruit cake, iced (100g)	65.9	1.3	64.6	3.6	9.8	350
Sponge, 16oz (¹/₁₂ cake)	23.2	0.2	23.0	2.1	1.0	110
Pie						
Apple, 23cm, frozen (¹/₈ pie)	42.5	2.0	40.5	2.4	13.8	296
Blueberry, 23cm, frozen (¹/₈ pie)	43.6	1.3	42.3	2.3	12.5	290
Cherry, 23cm, frozen (¹/₈ pie)	49.8	1.0	48.8	2.5	13.8	325
Coconut custard, 20cm (¹/₆ pie)	31.4	1.9	29.5	6.1	13.7	270
Lemon meringue, 23cm, homemade (¹/₈ pie)	49.7	1.5	48.1	4.8	16.4	362
Peach, 23cm, homemade (¹/₈ pie)	55.4	2.0	53.5	3.2	16.3	375
Pecan, 23cm, homemade (¹/₈ pie)	63.7	6.1	57.6	6.0	27.1	503
Pumpkin, 23cm, homemade (¹/₈ pie)	40.9	4.2	36.7	7.0	14.4	316
Rhubarb, 23cm (¹/₈ pie)	45.1	0.0	45.1	3.0	12.6	507

Food Item (Amount)	Carb (g)	Fibre (g)	Net Carbs (g)	Protein (g)	Fat (g)	Cals
Strawberry Cream Tart (1)	33.4	1.4	32.0	2.5	15.8	281
Pie Crust						
Pie crust, 23cm, frozen (1/8 pie)	7.9	0.2	7.8	0.7	5.3	82

SNACKS, BISCUITS AND SWEETS

Stick to controlled carb snacks and sweets and you'll do fine. Otherwise, it would be best to avoid foods in this category.

Food Item (Amount)	Carb (g)	Fibre (g)	Net Carbs (g)	Protein (g)	Fat (g)	Cals
Biscuits						
Chocolate chip cookies (100g)	65.2	2.0	63.2	5.8	22.9	474
Crunch creams (100g)	67.9	1.0	66.9	5.2	24.6	497
Digestives, choc (100g)	66.5	2.2	64.3	6.8	24.1	493
Digestives, plain (100g)	68.6	2.2	66.4	6.3	20.3	465
Flapjacks (100g)	62.4	2.6	59.8	4.8	27.0	493
Fig Rolls (2)	22.7	1.5	21.2	1.2	2.3	111
Gingernut (100g)	79.1	1.4	77.7	5.6	13.0	436
Ginger Snaps (2)	11.0	0.3	10.8	0.5	1.3	60
Hob Nobs (100g)	65.2	3.5	61.7	7.6	21.4	468
Oatmeal, 5cm (2)	20.9	1.2	19.7	2.4	6.2	148
Sandwich biscuits, cream-filled (100g)	72.5	1.6	70.9	5.9	20.7	482
Sandwich biscuits, jam-filled (100g)	69.5	1.5	68	5.6	17.3	439
Shortbread (2)	10.3	0.3	10.0	1.0	3.9	80
Sugar wafer with cream filling (2)	4.9	0.0	4.9	0.3	1.7	36
Vienna Fingers (2)	21.0	0.0	21.0	1.0	6.0	150
Walker's Shortbread (1)	11.0	0.0	11.0	1.0	6.0	100

Food Item (Amount)	Carb (g)	Fibre (g)	Net Carbs (g)	Protein (g)	Fat (g)	Cals
Sweets						
Boiled Sweets, all flavours (4 pieces)	23.5	0.0	23.5	0.0	0.1	95
Bounty bar (100g)	58.1	3.2	54.9	3.7	26.3	469
Cadbury Dairy (10 squares)	24.0	1.0	23.0	3.0	12.0	220
Cadbury Fruit and Nut (10 squares)	25.0	1.0	24.0	3.0	10.0	200
Caramel Twix (50g bar)	37.4	0.6	36.8	2.6	13.9	284
Galaxy milk chocolate	56.9	0.8	56.1	7.7	30.7	520
Gumdrops (10 pieces)	35.6	0.0	35.6	0.0	0.0	139
Jellybeans (10 pieces)	10.2	0.0	10.2	0.0	0.1	40
Kit Kat (15g)	26.9	0.8	26.1	3.0	10.7	216
M&M's Peanut (10 pieces)	12.1	0.7	11.4	1.9	5.3	103
M&M's Plain (20 pieces)	10.0	0.4	9.6	0.6	3.0	69
Mars bar (100g)	77.3	0.4	76.9	4.5	18.3	473
Milk chocolate (40g bar)	26.1	1.5	24.6	3.0	13.5	226
Milk chocolate w/almonds (40g bar)	21.8	2.5	19.3	3.7	14.1	216
Milky Way (50g bar)	43.0	1.0	42.0	2.7	9.7	254
Plain chocolate	63.5	2.5	61	5.0	28.0	510
Raisinets (20 pieces)	14.2	1.0	13.2	0.9	3.2	82
Snickers (50g bar)	33.8	1.4	32.3	4.6	14.0	273
Starburst Fruit Chews (5 pieces)	21.1	0.0	21.1	0.1	2.1	99
Sunmaid raisins (100g)	71.4	5.8	65.6	3.0	0.7	304
Twix	68.5	0.8	67.7	4.6	24.1	492

Food Item (Amount)	Carb (g)	Fibre (g)	Net Carbs (g)	Protein (g)	Fat (g)	Cals
Snacks, Savory						
Bombay Mix (100g)	35.1	6.2	28.9	18.8	32.9	503
CHEESE SNACKS						
Cheetos Crunchy (21 pieces)	15.0	1.0	14.0	2.0	10.0	160
Cheetos Curls (20 pieces)	20.0	1.3	18.7	2.7	13.3	200
CORN CHIPS						
Barbecue (20 pieces)	20.2	1.9	18.4	2.5	11.8	188
Fritos Original (20 pieces)	9.4	0.6	8.8	1.3	6.3	100
CRISPS						
Barbecue (20 pieces)	13.7	1.1	12.6	2.0	8.4	128
Potato crisps (100g)	53.3	5.3	48	5.7	34.2	530
Potato crisps lower fat (100g)	63.5	5.9	57.6	6.6	21.5	458
Pringles Original (14 pieces)	15.0	1.0	14.0	1.0	11.0	160
Onion rings, dry snack (25g)	19.5	0.0	19.5	0.1	6.0	134
Pork Scratchings (100g)	0.2	0.3	0.1	47.9	46.0	606
PRETZELS						
Rods (3 pieces)	22.0	1.0	21.0	3.0	1.0	110
Soft (1)	38.4	0.9	37.5	4.5	1.7	190
Sticks (45 pieces)	21.6	0.9	20.6	2.8	0.9	103
Twisted (5 pieces)	23.8	1.0	22.8	2.7	1.1	114
TORTILLA CHIPS						
Doritos 3D Cool Ranch (20 pieces)	13.3	0.7	12.6	1.5	4.4	104
Doritos Nacho Cheesier (20 pieces)	22.7	1.3	21.3	2.7	9.3	187
Tortilla chips (20 pieces)	22.6	2.3	20.3	2.5	9.4	180

Food Item (Amount)	Carb (g)	Fibre (g)	Net Carbs (g)	Protein (g)	Fat (g)	Cals
Twiglets (100g)	62.0	10.3	51.7	11.3	11.7	383
Wotsits (100g)	54.3	1.0	53.3	7.0	31.9	519

BAKING PRODUCTS

Refined flour is very high in carbohydrates, so stick to a combination of groundnuts, soya and other protein flours and specially designed products. Note that spices such as cinnamon and nutmeg are relatively high in carbs. When purchasing extracts, especially vanilla, be sure to look for natural flavours.

Food Item (Amount)	Carb (g)	Fibre (g)	Net Carbs (g)	Protein (g)	Fat (g)	Cals
Baking powder ($\frac{1}{2}$tsp)	0.0	0.0	0.0	0.0	0.0	0
Bicarbonate of soda ($\frac{1}{2}$tsp)	0.0	0.0	0.0	0.0	0.0	0
Chocolate, baking, unsweetened (25g)	8.0	4.4	3.7	2.9	15.7	148
Chocolate chips, semisweet (2tbs)	14.4	1.3	13.0	1.0	6.8	109
Chocolate chips, semisweet, mini (2tbs)	13.7	1.3	12.4	0.9	6.5	104
Cinnamon, ground (1tsp)	1.8	1.3	0.6	0.1	0.1	6
Cocoa powder, unsweetened (2tbs)	5.8	3.6	2.3	2.1	1.5	25
Coconut, desiccated (1tbs)	3.1	1.8	1.3	0.7	6.7	71
Coconut milk, tinned (120ml)	3.2	1.3	1.9	2.3	24.1	223
Cornmeal (2tbs)	13.4	1.3	12.1	1.5	0.3	63
Flour, plain (50g)	23.9	0.8	23.0	3.2	0.3	114
Gelatin, unsweetened (1 sachet)	0.0	0.0	0.0	6.0	0.0	23

Food Item (Amount)	Carb (g)	Fibre (g)	Net Carbs (g)	Protein (g)	Fat (g)	Cals
Ghee (1tsp)	0.0	0.0	0.0	0.0	4.3	37
Treacle (1tbs)	14.1	0.0	14.1	0.0	0.0	55
Sugar, brown (1tsp)	4.5	0.0	4.5	0.0	0.0	17
Sugar, white (1tsp)	4.2	0.0	4.2	0.0	0.0	16

Dining Out

When watching your carb intake, it's easier to choose wisely in restaurants where familiar dishes are served. Ethnic restaurants present more of a challenge because food combinations, typical dishes and, often, ingredients are different. (Of course, that's why we opt for ethnic cuisines in the first place!) The charts that follow will help you make smarter choices. We've given guidelines rather than carb counts because recipes and portion sizes vary greatly from restaurant to restaurant.

General Guidelines

• Don't arrive at a restaurant starving – it makes the contents of the breadbasket irresistible. To blunt your appetite, eat a hard-boiled egg or a few slices of cheese before you go out.

• Many restaurants feature their menus on-line. If possible, visit the website ahead of time to see if there are appropriate options and decide what you will order.

• Ask your waiter or waitress to explain any menu listings you don't understand. And keep in mind that most restaurants will substitute a portion of vegetables for potatoes, rice or pasta upon request.

• Ask for sauces on the side so that you can decide whether and how much to consume.

• Start your meal with a soup or salad – it will help fill you up. Likewise, drink plenty of water before your meal.

• Don't torture yourself if you accidentally consume something that's been batter dipped or breaded. Remember, it's only one meal.

• As far as dessert goes, you have two choices if you are beyond the Induction phase: fruit with unsweetened whipped cream or a golf-ball-sized portion of a 'regular dessert'. Otherwise, skip dessert – until you get home and can indulge in a controlled carb treat.

In Chinese Restaurants

Choose . . .	Instead of . . .
Egg Drop Soup	Egg Rolls
Shrimp Sizzling Platter	Shrimp Fried Rice
Steamed Tofu (bean curd) with Vegetables	Any Chow Fun (wide noodle) dish
Stir-Fried Pork with Garlic Sauce	Sweet and Sour Pork
Beef with Chinese Mushrooms	Any Lo Mein (narrow noodle) dish
Steamed Whole Fish (Sea Bass)	Shrimp with Black Bean Sauce
Chicken with Walnuts	Chicken with Cashews
Sautéed Spinach with Garlic	Moo Shu Vegetables (with pancakes)

Note:

If you're on Induction, stick to dishes that are stir-fried, steamed or grilled, and ask for sauces to be served on the side. On Ongoing Weight Loss, choose one sauced dish and one simply prepared dish. By the time you are on Pre-Maintenance and Lifetime Maintenance – and if your metabolism allows it – you may enjoy 100–225g (uncooked weight) of brown rice with your meal.

In French Restaurants

Choose . . .	Instead of . . .
Frisée Salad with Lardons (thin strips of bacon) and Poached Egg	Quiche Lorraine (bacon, onion and egg pie)
Coquilles St Jacques (scallops in cream sauce with cheese)	Langoustine en Croûte (lobster in puff pastry)
Moules Marinière (mussels in white wine and herbs) or Bouillabaisse (fish stew)	Vichyssoise (cream of leek and potato soup)
Coq au Vin (chicken in wine sauce)	Canard a l'Orange or aux Cerises (duck with orange sauce or cherry sauce)
Entrecôte or Tournedos Bordelaise (steak in reduced shallot and red wine sauce)	Croque Monsieur (egg-dipped fried ham and egg sandwich)
Veal Marengo (veal stew with tomatoes and mushrooms)	Veal Prince Orloff (veal roast stuffed with rice, onions and mushrooms)

Haricots Verts au Beurre (buttered young green beans)

Assorted cheese plate

Pommes Anna (upside-down potato cake)

Crepes Suzette (crepes with orange butter and orange liqueur, served flambéed)

Note:

Southern French cooking, as well as bistro food, generally offers a wider range of choices than classic French cuisine because the preparations are simpler. In classic French, opt for beurre blanc sauces instead of béchamel sauces because the latter contain flour. And beware of *pommes frites* (chips), which tend to arrive in heaps with steak dishes.

In Greek Restaurants

Choose . . .	Instead of . . .
Tsatziki (yogurt and cucumber dip)	Skordalia (potato and garlic dip)
Avgolemono (chicken soup with egg and lemon)	Spanakopita (spinach and cheese pie)
Taramosalata (fish roe dip)	Dolmades (rice stuffed vine leaves)
Beef or Lamb Souvlaki (marinated, then charcoal grilled)	Moussaka (fried aubergine layered with meat and white sauces)
Roast Leg of Lamb, Grilled Lamb Chops or Braised Lamb Shanks	Pastitsio (casserole layered with pasta, meat and white sauce)

Chicken Char-grilled with Lemon, Garlic and Oregano or Rosemary	Chicken Pilaf
Braised Pork Loin with Lemon and Fennel	Any potato dish
Char-grilled Prawns, Octopus or Swordfish	Fried Kalamari (squid)

Note:

Instead of using pitta bread for dipping into *tsatziki* or *taramosalata*, ask for raw veggies. A good dessert option in Greek restaurants is a cheese platter. Cheese such as Kasseri, haloumi and mizithra offer a variety of textures and flavours.

In Italian Restaurants

Choose . . .	Instead of . . .
Insalata frutti di mare (seafood salad)	Fried Calamari
Mixed Char-grilled Vegetables or Sautéed Portabello Mushrooms	Fried, Breaded Mozzarella (Mozzarella in Carozza)
Rocket and Fennel Salad with Parmesan Shavings	Prosciutto with Melon
Antipasto (assorted meats and cheeses), Marinated Peppers and Mushrooms, Clams	Baked Stuffed Clams (usually breadcrumb heavy)
Escarole or Stracciatella (broth and egg drop) soup	Fettuccine Alfredo

Roasted Red Snapper or Salmon;
Char-grilled Calamari, Shrimp
or Scampi

Linguine with Clam Sauce

Char-grilled Chicken Paillard
(boneless breast, pounded thin)
or Pork Loin

Any risotto (creamy rice
dishes)

Veal or Chicken Piccata or
Scaloppini (very thin veal or
chicken fillets with lemon
and capers)

Veal or Chicken Parmesan

Note:

Instead of nibbling bread while you peruse the menu, eat a few olives instead. And do as the Italians do: start your meal with a bowl of soup (see choices above); it will help fill you up. The carb grams in tomato sauces vary widely, and can be quite high, so use your judgement: if a dish is buried in sauce, gently push some to the side.

In Indian Restaurants
Choose . . .

Shahi Paneer (homemade cheese
in creamy tomato sauce)

Roasted Aubergine with Onions
and Spices

Chicken Shorba Soup (made
with garlic, ginger, cinnamon
and spices)

Instead of . . .

Vegetable Samosas
(pastries)

Any Pakora (fritter)

Lentil or Mulligatawny
Soup

Any Korma (meat in cream sauce)

Any Biryani (rice dish)

Any Tandoori (oven roasted)

Any Pilaf (rice dish)

Lamb or Chicken Curry

Any Dal (lentil or bean dish)

Any Lamb, Chicken or Shrimp Kebab

Lamb, Chicken or Shrimp Saag (cooked with spinach and spices)

Note:

To start your meal, request some spiced cooked vegetables or a cooked cheese dish, such as the Shahi Paneer (see chart). Enquire about all the ingredients in a specific dish because Indian food combines so many that menus do not list them all. 'Vindaloo' dishes, which are very spicy curries, often contain potatoes.

In Japanese Restaurants Choose . . .

Instead of . . .

Oshinko (pickled vegetables)

Okonomiyaki (pancake-pizza)

Steamed Broccoli or Mixed Vegetables (no sauce), or Char-grilled Aubergine

Gyoza (fried vegetable dumplings)

Sashimi (raw fish without rice)

Sushi (raw fish with rice)

Shabu Shabu (meat and vegetables in broth)

Tonkatsu (deep-fried pork)

Grilled Sea Bass (or any grilled fish of the day), soy or ginger sauce only

Miso (soya bean paste) soup

Negamaki (green onions wrapped in paper-thin slices of beef)

Shrimp Tempura (batter-fried shrimp)

Seafood Soba or Udon (noodle soups)

Beef Teriyaki

Note:

Seaweed salad is a pleasant and mild-tasting accompaniment to Japanese food, so try it (even if the ingredient is initially off-putting). Teriyaki sauce is sweetened with either corn syrup or sugar, so opt for plain soy sauce instead. Sip plenty of anti-oxidant-rich green tea with your meal. Its subtle flavour is best savoured on its own, without sugar substitute.

Fast Food

Keep in mind that much fast food is highly processed, loaded with carbohydrates and often prepared with trans fats (hydrogenated oils). But sometimes, eating in fast-food restaurants is unavoidable when you're on the go or don't want to make your friends or co-workers feel uncomfortable with your commitment to eating the controlled carb way. The fact is, you may end up in burger joints or pizza places from time to time, so when you're in such a place, you should know how to choose the most nutritionally sound meal options.

To make things easy for you, we've reviewed menus from top quick-service chains, assembled lists of popular items and put the best possible choices in boldface type. We've also listed menu items that are higher in carbohydrate so that you can see the vast difference in carb count between high- and lower-carb options. In some cases, you can 'remodel' a fast-food meal to reduce its carb count. For example, eating a burger without its bun can strip 29 grams of carbs off the tally. Although space does not allow us to include the full array of fast-food companies, armed with the information provided, you should be able to 'guesstimate' items at other chains. You can also check out their websites.

The nutritional analyses in this chapter come from the websites for included chain restaurants. In some cases, when we've 'remodelled' an item, such as removing the bun from a sandwich, we've estimated carb counts – we've double-starred those items.

Burger Chains

At a burger chain, go with the flow and have a beef patty sandwich. Yes, even a bacon cheeseburger! Just discard the bun and be sure to order the burger 'your way'. Mayonnaise and mustard are permissible but watch the ketchup, which is often full of sugar. Watch out, too, for special sauces, as sugar often lurks in them as well. Slices of tomato and lettuce garnish are fine. Steer clear of anything advertised as 'low fat' because this label often translates to high carb. Also, make sure you avoid chicken sandwiches if they're breaded and fried. Salads are usually a sensible choice (but go easy on fast-food salad dressings – most contain sugar or high-fructose corn syrup, so make sure you read labels on the packets).

Food Item (Amount)	Carb (g)	Fibre (g)	Net Carbs (g)	Protein (g)	Fat (g)	Cals
McDonald's						
www.mcdonalds.com						
Cheeseburger (1)	36.0	2.0	34.0	15.0	14.0	330
Big Mac® (1)	47.0	3.0	44.0	24.0	34.0	590
**Hamburger patty (1)	0.0	N/a	0.0	12.0	12.0	110
Chicken McGrill® Sandwich (1)	46.0	2.0	44.0	26.0	18.0	450

**estimated carb counts

Food Item (Amount)	Carb (g)	Fibre (g)	Net Carbs (g)	Protein (g)	Fat (g)	Cals
¨Chicken Fillet (1)	4.0	N/a	4.0	21.0	4.5	35
McSalad Shaker® Salads						
Chef Salad (1)	5.0	2.0	3.0	17.0	8.0	150
Garden Salad (1)	4.0	2.0	2.0	7.0	6.0	100
Burger King						
www.bk.com						
Hamburger (1)	30.0	2.0	28.0	18.0	14.0	130
Hamburger patty (1)	0.0	0.0	0.0	11.0	10.0	140
Whopper® (1)	53.0	4.0	49.0	29.0	39.0	680
Whopper® Patty (1)	0.0	0.0	0.0	25.0	23.0	320
BK Broiler® Sandwich (1)	52.0	3.0	49.0	30.0	25.0	550
BK Broiler® chicken breast patty (1)	4.0	N/a	4.0	21.0	4.5	35
Wendy's®						
www.wendys.com						
Classic Single® with Everything (1)	37.0	3.0	34.0	25.0	19.0	410
100g Hamburger Patty (1)	0.0	0.0	0.0	19.0	14.0	200
50g Hamburger Patty (1)	0.0	0.0	0.0	9.0	7.0	100
Chicken Fillet Sandwich (1)	46.0	2.0	44.0	27.0	16.0	430
Grilled Chicken Fillet (1)	1.0	0.0	1.0	19.0	3.5	110

¨estimated carb counts

Pizza Chains

The bad news is you'll have to forgo the pizza. The good news, however, is that many major pizza chains serve chicken wings that are relatively low in carbs. Order the wings, visit the salad bar and you've got yourself a meal. Select acceptable vegetables as a salad base, then top with protein foods such as hard-boiled eggs, turkey or chicken. Avoid coleslaw, which may contain sugar, and pass up that pasta salad. Use oil and regular red- or white-wine vinegar instead of a prepared dressing; commercial dressings often contain sugar, and even balsamic vinegar has a smidgeon of sugar in it.

Baked stuffed potatoes are an absolute no-no. If it's absolutely necessary to order a pizza, eat only the cheese and fixings and leave the crust. It's a messy solution, but you'll avoid the nutrient-deficient high-carb crust.

Food Item (Amount)	Carb (g)	Fibre (g)	Net Carbs (g)	Protein (g)	Fat (g)	Cals
Pizza Hut®						
www.pizzahut.com						
Mild Buffalo Wings (5 pieces)	<1.0	0.0	<1.0	23.0	12.0	220
Hot Buffalo Wings (4 pieces)	4.0	1.0	3.0	22.0	12.0	210
Pepperoni Lover's® Pizza (1 slice)	27.0	2.0	25.0	11.0	11.0	250
Veggie Lover's® Pizza (1 slice)	29.0	2.0	27.0	9.0	8.0	220

Food Item (Amount)	Carb (g)	Fibre (g)	Net Carbs (g)	Protein (g)	Fat (g)	Cals
Domino's®						
www.dominos.com						
Buffalo Wings, BBQ						
(1 avg. piece)	1.5	<1.0	1.5	5.5	2.5	51
¨Buffalo Wings, hot						
(1 avg. piece)	0.5	<1.0	0.5	5.5	2.5	45
Classic Hand Tossed Pizza						
(¹/₄ of 30 cm medium pizza)	55.0	3.0	52.0	15.5	11.0	375
Crunchy Thin Crust						
(¹/₄ of 30cm medium pizza)	31.0	2.0	29.0	12.0	12.0	273
Ultimate Deep Dish						
(¹/₄ of 30cm medium pizza)	68.5	4.0	64.5	23.0	27.5	598

¨estimated carb counts

Chicken Chains

Here the challenge is to avoid anything that is bart[...]
breaded. Barbecue sauce is typically full of sugar, and s[...]
has probably seeped into the meat. The safest thing is to remove
the skin. Dry-rubbed meats are fine, or look for roasted chicken
and acceptable side dishes, such as salad. If there's a grilled-
chicken fillet sandwich available, grab it! Discard the bun, and
you've got a pretty good selection. Or, if necessary, scrape the
breading off a fried chicken breast.

NOTE: At KFC, it's better to scrape the breading off an
'Original Recipe' chicken breast than a 'Hot & Spicy' one – the
total carb count will be lower.

Food Item (Amount)	Carb (g)	Fibre (g)	Net Carbs (g)	Protein (g)	Fat (g)	Cals
KFC®						
www.kfc.com						
Original Recipe® Chicken						
Breast Sandwich (1)	16.0	1.0	15.0	29.0	24.0	400
Hot & Spicy Chicken						
Breast Sandwich (1)	23.0	1.0	22.0	38.0	29.0	505
Tender Roast® Sandwich						
w/out sauce (1)	23.0	1.0	22.0	31.0	5.0	270